Radiology and Imaging for Medical Students

Radiology and Imaging for Medical Students

David Sutton
MD FRCP FRCR DMRD MCAR(Hon)
Consulting Radiologist, St Mary's Hospital, London
Consulting Radiologist, National Hospitals for Neurology and Neurosurgery
(Queen Square and Maida Vale), London

SIXTH EDITION

CHURCHILL LIVINGSTONE
EDINBURGH LONDON MADRID MELBOURNE NEW YORK AND
TOKYO 1994

CHURCHILL LIVINGSTONE
Medical Division of Longman Group Limited

Distributed in the United States of America by Churchill
Livingstone Inc., 650 Avenue of the Americas, New York,
N.Y. 10011, and by associated companies, branches and
representatives throughout the world.

First edition 1965
Second edition 1971
Third edition 1977
Fourth edition 1982
Fifth edition 1988
Sixth edition 1994
Reprinted 1994
Reprinted 1995

ISBN 0 443 04883 5

British Library Cataloguing in Publication Data
A catalogue record for this book is available from the British
Library.

Library of Congress Cataloging in Publication Data
Sutton, David,
    Radiology and imaging for medical students/David Sutton.
    — 6th ed.
        p. cm.
    Includes index.
    ISBN 0-443-04883-5
    1. Diagnosis, Radioscopic. 2. Diagnostic imaging. I. Title.
    [DNLM: 1. Diagnostic Imaging.   WN 100 S967r 1994]
RC78.S88   1994
616.07′57—dc20
DNLM/DLC
for Library of Congress   93-19864

The
publisher's
policy is to use
paper manufactured
from sustainable forests

Printed in Hong Kong
WC/03

Contents

Preface

Roentgen discovered X-rays in December 1895 and the centenary of this remarkable discovery will occur shortly. For most of the last century X-rays remained the basic and only method of medical imaging. In the last three decades, however, there have been remarkable advances. Radioisotopes, ultrasound, computed tomography, and finally nuclear magnetic resonance have all become part of the radiologist's armoury and the Department of Radiology is now more appropriately called the Department of Medical Imaging. Modern high technology apparatus is now largely computer based and most equipment is now both complex and expensive.

Students need not be intimidated by this growth of complex and sophisticated machinery as long as they remember that the basic purpose is to demonstrate human anatomy and pathology affecting internal organs. In this Student's text the aim is to explain in the simplest terms the basic technical and physical principles of apparatus, and to show how the different methods are used in clinical practice to demonstrate the different internal organs and their diseases. They should also realise that this is a rapidly changing field in which new methods are constantly evolving and in which recent as well as long-established techniques can rapidly become obsolete.

David Sutton

Acknowledgements

Acknowledgements are gratefully made to the following colleagues for illustrations taken from *A Textbook of Radiology and Imaging*, 4th and 5th editions, edited by David Sutton: Dr Robert Dick, Dr Huw Gravelle, Dr J. H. Highman, Dr Ivan Hyde, Professor E. Rhys Davies, Professor Ian Isherwood, Dr Jeremy P. R. Jenkins, Dr Brian Kendall, Dr W. R. Lees, Dr Peter Phelps, Dr Richard Mason, Dr Janet Murfitt, Dr Maurice Raphael, Dr Frank Ross, Dr Michael Rubens, Dr Keith Simpkins, Dr Gordon Thomson.

1. Introduction

Modern imaging departments use a variety of different techniques to provide images of human internal organs and to demonstrate pathological lesions within them. These techniques can be classified as:

1. Methods using ionising radiation
   a. Simple X-rays
   b. Computed X-ray tomography – generally referred to as computed tomography or CT
   c. Radioisotope scanning – also referred to as nuclear medicine, radionuclide scanning or scintiscanning.
2. Other methods
   a. Ultrasound
   b. Magnetic resonance imaging (MRI).

Ionising radiation in large doses has well-known dangers, including carcinogenesis and local tissue damage, but the amounts used in modern imaging practice are minimal and innocuous.

X-rays were discovered in 1895 by Conrad Roentgen who was then an obscure German physicist. For some 60 years (until the middle of this century) they provided the only practical method of medical imaging. Isotope scanning was introduced into medical practice in the 1950s and ultrasound in the 1960s. CT was developed in the 1970s and MRI in the 1980s. All these methods advanced rapidly and are now important subspecialties in their own right.

X-rays

X-rays are part of the so-called electro-magnetic spectrum (Fig. 1.1). These range from wireless waves at the long end of the spectrum to cosmic rays at the short end. Because of their short

1

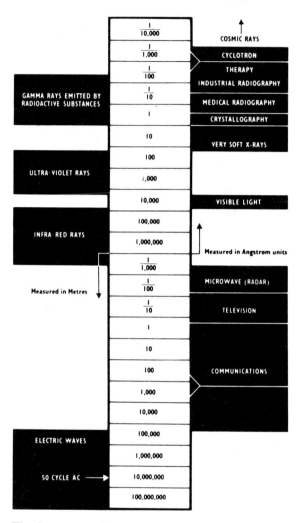

Fig. 1.1 The electro-magnetic spectrum.

wavelength X-rays can penetrate materials which do not transmit visible light. Roentgen's discovery was the starting point for modern medical radiology and radiotherapy and for many other non-medical sciences which have developed over the years from the use of X-rays. Modern X-ray apparatus is highly sophisticated but the method of producing X-rays remains basically the same as that used by Roentgen himself. High voltage electric current is passed across a vacuum tube. This induces a stream of electrons from an electrically heated metal element (cathode) to strike a metal target (anode) after passing across the vacuum. When the beam of electrons strikes the anode X-rays are produced (Fig. 1.2).

Methods of X-ray examination

1. *Simple radiography* is the method in which an X-ray beam is passed through the patient on to a photographic plate (Fig. 1.3). It has been practised continuously since Roentgen's original discovery. Modern sophisticated apparatus can produce films with exposures taken within 0.1 of a second or less.

2. *Tomography* has been in use for over seventy years but again the method has been steadily improved by technical advances so that today it is possible to demonstrate detail of the inner ear by this

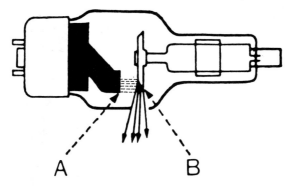

A   **B**

Fig. 1.2 Diagram of a modern rotating anode X-ray tube. Electrons at high KV travel across the vacuum from the cathode (A) to the rotating anode (B) to generate the X-rays (shown as arrows emerging from tube).

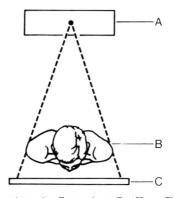

Fig. 1.3 Simple X-ray: A = tube; B = patient; C = X-ray film.

technique, including the ossicles. Tomography is a variation of the simple X-ray film method which permits tissue section radiographs to be obtained. During the X-ray exposure the X-ray tube and the X-ray film are moved in opposite directions so as to produce the equivalent of a body section X-ray. The technique is now mainly used in chest work, but is also used in bone work and in other areas.

Figure 1.4 illustrates the basic technique of tomography. As the tube moves in one direction the film moves in the opposite direction. The two are connected by a rod which can be made to pivot at variable point A. Since A remains stationary during the whole procedure the part of the body in line with A is the only part which will be clearly shown. Several films can be taken at the same time by the use of the so-called multi-section box. Thus multiple body sections can be obtained with a single exposure. Modern apparatus includes specialised tomographic equipment of *rotatory* and *epicyclic* movement.

3. *Screening and the image intensifier.* Screening is the term used for passing an X-ray beam through the patient to impinge on a fluorescent screen. In the past (before 1950) the fluorescent image thus produced was observed from the opposite side of the screen by a radiologist (Fig. 1.5). A darkened room and dark adaptation by the radiologist were necessary, because the brightness of the image was inadequate for daylight viewing. The development of the image intensifier in the 1950s rendered this simple method obsolete. With the image intensifier the fluorescent screen is viewed through an electronic intensifier and then passed through television cameras to a monitor in a closed circuit television (Fig. 1.6). The monitor is observed by the radiologist. Screening with the image

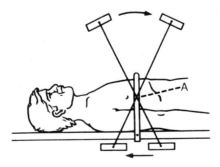

Fig. 1.4   Diagram to illustrate tomography: A = pivot point of bar connecting tube and films.

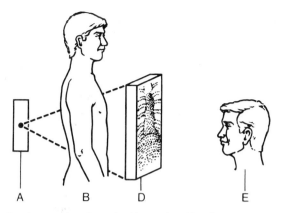

Fig. 1.5 Simple screening: A = tube; B = patient; D = fluorescent screen; E = radiologist.

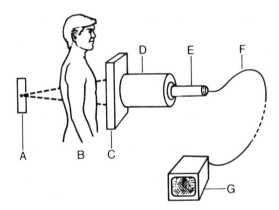

Fig. 1.6 Screening with image intensifier and television link: A = tube; B = patient; C = fluorescent screen; D = image intensifier; A = television camera; F = closed circuit to television monitor; G = television monitor.

intensifier can be recorded on cinefilm or a video tape machine and recordings played back at the convenience of the operator. The images can also be recorded on cut film or roll film.

4. *Cineradiography.* As already mentioned, the brightened image produced by an image intensifier can be utilised for cineradiography. The cine camera is usually attached to the image intensifier in place of the television camera shown in Figure 1.6. The method is particularly useful for studying disorders of swallowing (barium swallow) and for coronary angiography and left ventricular angiocardiography.

5. *Miniature radiography.* This method was once widely used in the form of 'mass miniature radiography'. Since X-rays, unlike light rays, cannot be focused or bent by lenses, miniatures can only be obtained by taking optical photographs of a fluorescent image obtained as described in (3) above. Such miniature films are very much cheaper than conventional X-ray films. Large populations have been rapidly screened by using a 70 mm or 100 mm roll film camera to photograph the chest images of patients standing consecutively before a screening stand. The method however, involves five or six times the radiation dosage of a conventional X-ray film. In this country, therefore, where the pick-up rate for tuberculosis has become negligible, the method has fallen into disuse as a screening procedure.

The method is also used via the image intensifier as a cheaper method of recording such screening examinations as barium meals. There is a considerable cost saving in recording a barium examination on 100 mm film rather than on conventional large films.

6. *Xeroradiography.* An aluminium plate is coated with a thin layer of selenium and charged electrically. An X-ray beam is passed through the patient on to the plate and this causes an alteration of the electrostatic charge corresponding with the image. The image can be shown by blowing a thin powder, which adheres in proportion to the local charge, on to the plate. This is transferred to special paper and a permanent record obtained.

The advantage of xeroradiography is that it provides soft tissue contrast of sensitivity not obtainable with conventional film. So far the method has been most widely used in *mammography* for the demonstration of breast tumours (see Ch. 13).

7. *Digital vascular imaging* (DVI) uses image intensifier screening as described above to obtain images of blood vessels. Preliminary screening of the area to be examined is followed immediately by screening as a bolus of contrast material injected intravenously or intra-arterially passes through the blood vessels. The preliminary images can be electronically subtracted from the images with contrast medium. This leaves a clear bone free image of the blood vessels which is recorded on cut film. The technique is also referred to as digital subtraction angiography (DSA), and is illustrated in Chapters 4 and 12.

8. *Special techniques and procedures using X-rays.* A wide variety of specialised techniques using X-rays is available to the Radiologist. These range from relatively simple and innocuous examinations such as barium meals to complicated and potentially dangerous

procedures such as cerebral and coronary angiography which may require general anaesthesia. These techniques are discussed in the appropriate systemic chapters.

Contrast media

Radiology makes great use of media which have a different permeability to X-rays than that of the body. These can be inserted into various cavities and organs, or even into blood vessels or arteries. As a result it is possible to obtain X-ray pictures of the interior of organs or blood vessels. The contrast media generally used are:

1. *Salts of heavy metals.* Barium is the heavy metal most widely used in radiology. As barium sulphate it has long been used for gastro-intestinal work, both for barium meals and for barium enemas. Proprietary preparations have come into general usage (e.g. Micropaque) which have special properties allowing the barium to produce better coating of the mucosa.

Sodium iodide has been used as a contrast medium in the past, mainly for cystography.

2. *Organic iodide preparations.* These were originally introduced for the demonstration of the *urinary tract* in forms which were excreted by the kidneys after intravenous injection. They were also used for the demonstration of the *gall-bladder* in a form which could be taken orally, absorbed from the intestines, and then excreted in the liver. Recent decades have witnessed a steady increase and improvement in the types of organic iodides available both for pyelography and for cholecystography. These will be described and discussed later. The organic iodides which are injected intravenously for pyelograms also became widely used for *angiocardiography, arteriography* and *phlebography.* Advances in this field have been rapid and several newer and safer contrast media have been introduced in the past decade. Water soluble organic iodide media are also used for *myelography,* e.g. iopamidol.

3. *Gas.* Air and other gases are completely permeable to X-rays and appear on film as negative or black compared to the positive or white appearance of radiopaque substances such as bone, or the varying shades of grey produced by soft tissues. Air is normally present in the lungs and respiratory passages, in the pharynx and paranasal sinuses, and in more or less degree in the alimentary tract. In all these areas its negative shadow is readily recognised and made use of.

Air can be used together with barium for so-called 'double contrast' studies of both the colon and the stomach. The barium coats the mucosa which can be shown and studied in detail following air distension of the viscus. It has also been used in the bladder for double contrast cystography and in joints for arthrography.

In the past it was widely used in the CNS for encephalography and ventriculography but these procedures were rendered obsolete with the advent of CT and MRI.

Interventional radiology

In recent decades radiodiagnostic techniques have been increasingly used for therapy as well as for diagnosis. So-called *interventional radiology* now involves a wide variety of procedures. These include:

1. Percutaneous catheterisation and embolisation in the treatment of tumours; this is mainly to reduce their size and vascularity prior to operation in difficult cases, or as a palliative measure in inoperable tumours. Percutaneous catheterisation and embolisation is also used for treatment of internal haemorrhage and for the treatment of angiomas and arteriovenous fistulae.

2. Percutaneous catheterisation with balloon catheters can be used to occlude arteries temporarily, either to stop haemorrhage or to obtain a bloodless field at operation.

3. Percutaneous catheterisation is also used for the delivery of chemotherapeutic drugs to tumours, or for the delivery of vasospastic drugs in patients with internal haemorrhage. It is also used for thrombolysis by delivering thrombolytic drugs directly to the clot.

4. Percutaneous transluminal dilatation of arterial stenoses is now being practised for the treatment of localised stenoses in the femoral and iliac arteries. The method has been extended to many other arterier including the renal artery and the coronary arteries.

5. Needle biopsy under imaging control is widely practised both for lung tumours and abdominal masses of all kinds.

6. Transhepatic catheterisation of the portal vein and embolisation of varices.

7. Transhepatic catheterisation of the bile ducts both for drainage in obstructive jaundice and for dilatation of stenosing strictures or insertion of prostheses.

8. Needle puncture and drainage of cysts in the kidney or other organs using control by simple X-ray or ultrasound.

9. Percutaneous catheterisation of the renal pelvis for antegrade pyelography or hydronephrosis drainage.

10. Percutaneous removal of residual biliary duct stones through the 'T' tube tract.

11. Percutaneous catheterisation and drainage of intra-abdominal abscesses.

This list will no doubt be further extended in the future and is discussed in detail in Chapter 13.

Examining an X-ray film

The student should develop as a routine a systematic approach to the examination of any X-ray film. The technique is described in detail in Chapter 2 (see p. 21), but the same principles of a routine systematic approach should be applied to the examination of any film, whether of chest, abdomen, skull, spine or limb.

Computed tomography

A new method of forming images from X-rays was developed and introduced into clinical use by a British physicist Godfrey Hounsfield in 1972. This is now usually referred to as computed tomography (CT) or computerised axial tomography (CAT). This was the greatest step forward in radiology since the discovery of X-rays by Roentgen in 1895. Hounsfield was awarded the Nobel Prize for medicine jointly with Professor A. N. Cormack in 1979. The principle of CT scanning is that conventional X-ray films provide only a small proportion of the data theoretically available when X-rays are passed through human tissues. By using multi-directional scanning of the patient, multiple data are collected concerning all tissues in the path of the X-ray beams. The X-rays fall not on the X-ray film but on to detectors which convert X-ray photons into scintillations. The detector response is directly related to the number of photons impinging on it and so to tissue density since more X-ray photons are absorbed by denser tissues. The scintillations produced can be quantified and recorded digitally. The information is fed into a computer which produces different readings as the X-ray beam traverses round the patient. The computer is required to deal with a vast number of digital readings. These can be presented as a numerical read-out representing the X-ray absorption in each tiny segment of tissue traversed. The information can also be presented in analogue form as a two-dimensional display of the matrix on a screen where each numerical value is represented by a single picture element (pixel).

The first machine had only two detectors and housed a sharply collimated beam of X-rays. The more modern machines use a fan beam and multiple detectors (Fig. 1.7). The early machines were used for head scanning only but these were superseded by 'body scanners' which can examine all parts of the body including the head. The original machines took 4½ minutes to perform a single tomographic slice but the present generation of machines can obtain scans in times varying from one to ten seconds according to type.

Data presentation

The analogue images are presented on a cathode ray tube immediately after each section. The picture is usually in grey scale in which the more radiopaque tissue, e.g. bone, appears white and the more radiolucent tissue appears in shades of grey. The range can be varied by changing the gate or window width (W) at will so that the tissues can be evaluated within a wide or narrow range of density. The central point or level (L) of the window can also be varied. The Hounsfield scale is used by most machines in which the fixed points are water at 0 and air at –1000, and dense bones at +1000. Figure 1.8 illustrates the scale and also the expanded central segment which contains most normal tissues.

Radioisotope scanning

Isotopes of an element are nuclides with the same atomic number

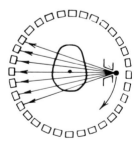

Fig. 1.7   Diagram showing relationship of X-ray tube and ring of detectors in a modern CT body scanner. The tube rotates around the patient. The detectors remain stationary.

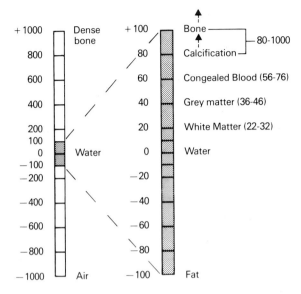

Fig. 1.8 Hounsfield's scale. The full scale on the left extends over 2000 units. The expanded scale on the right extends over 200 units and includes all body tissues. Head scans are usually done routinely at a window level (L) of 34–40 and a window (W) covering 0–75.

and therefore the same chemical and biological behaviour but with a different mass number and often a different energy state, e.g. the isotopes of iodine are ^{123}I, ^{125}I, and ^{131}I.

Radionuclides and *radioisotopes* are radioactive varieties but the terms in practice are interchangeable with nuclides and isotopes. Most of them are made artificially and disintegrate spontaneously, emitting radiation which includes gamma radiation. This is an electro-magnetic wave radiation of high penetrating power. The energy is measured in electron-Volts (eV).

The *half-life* of a radioisotope is the time taken for its activity to fall by one half, e.g 6 hours for technetium (^{99}Tc^{m}).

Almost every organ of the body can be investigated by means of radioisotope scanning. It is important, however, that the radiation dose to the patient should be kept to the minimum by using low doses of substances with short half-lives.

Technique of scanning

The technique of scanning depends on the fact that particular isotopes can be so designed as to be selectively taken up by particular organs.

In the individual organ, lesions such as tumours may take up selectively more of the isotope resulting in so-called 'hot' areas on the scan, as in the brain. Alternatively, they may fail to take up the isotope resulting in 'cold' areas, as in the liver. The uptake can be recorded as an 'image' by scanning machines.

Basically, a scanning machine consists of a *detector*. This is usually a large crystal of sodium iodide containing thallium iodide as activator. Gamma rays emitted by the isotope and striking the detector are converted directly into light quanta or photons. These are led off into a photomultiplier. This converts the light quanta into a small voltage pulse and the number of pulses is directly related to the original radioactivity.

The gamma camera. The gamma camera is more flexible than the earlier linear, scanner. It has a large stationary crystal which records activity over the whole of its field at the same time. The size of the field is limited by the size of the crystal but the whole field can be shown as an image on a cathode-ray tube and the image can then be photographed with a camera.

Since the activity recorded by the scanners is converted into electrical pulses, these can be recorded in digital form. This digital information can be fed into a computer and manipulated to provide physiological information about what is happening in the particular organ (data processing).

Ultrasound

Ultrasonic diagnosis employs sound waves whose frequency is far higher than can be registered by the human ear. These ultrasonic waves are produced from a transducer and travel through human tissues at a velocity of some 1500 metres per second. When the wave reaches an object or surface with a different texture, or acoustic nature, a wave is reflected back. These echoes are received by the apparatus and changed into electric current. This can be amplified and shown on a cathode-ray tube.

Transducers are substances that have the property of being able to convert one form of energy into another. Ultrasound transducers are made of materials that are mechanically deformed when an electric voltage is applied to them. This is the direct 'piezo-electric' (pressure electric) effect. Conversely if mechanical stress is applied voltage is generated (converse piezo-electric effect). The substance most widely used in medical ultrasonics is lead zirconate titanate (Fig. 1.9). In practice several forms of echo sounding display are available. These include:

A-scope. This was one of the early forms of clinical ultrasound. Using a single stationary probe the ultrasound reflections are recorded on an oscilloscope and appear as variations in amplitude. It enables linear measurements to be made between internal structures and was once widely used for measurement of displacement of the midline structures of the brain.

B-scope. With this method echoes are shown, not as deflections of varying amplitude, but as dots of varying brightness. As the transducer moves over the skin the series of linear dots are frozen as bright lines which form a two-dimensional image representing a linear section of the organ under examination. Grey-scale is a further refinement enabling the B-scan to be sealed in varying shades of grey to give a more realistic picture.

M-mode. It this technique a linear scan is held whilst a time-position graph of any motion builds up. Moving points are seen to oscillate forming wavy lines whilst stationary parts are represented as straight lines. In this way a time-position graph of moving parts is built up. The method proved most valuable in cardiac work,

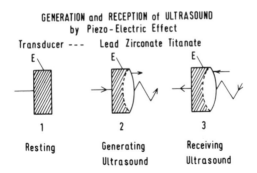

GENERATION and RECEPTION of ULTRASOUND
by Piezo-Electric Effect

Transducer --- Lead Zirconate Titanate

1
Resting

2
Generating
Ultrasound

3
Receiving
Ultrasound

Fig. 1.9 Generation and reception of ultrasound. 1. The transducer (hatched) coated with conducting material is in a resting phase. 2. A voltage (→) is applied to the transducer surface. The transducer resonates in response and it produces ultrasound from its surface (∧∧) (direct piezo-electric effect). 3. A pulse of ultrasound (∧∨) strikes the surface of the transducer which resonates as a result. A voltage (←) is generated on the transducer surface (converse piezo-electric effect).

particularly in the assessment of valvular lesions (Figs 1.10 and 1.11) but is now largely superseded.

Real time two dimensional scanning is a further advance on the B-scan in which an automatic scanning mechanism is used to pro-

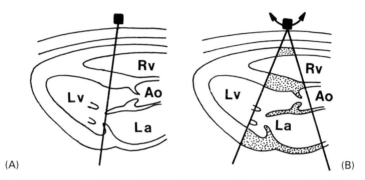

(A)   (B)

Fig. 1.10 (A) shows single static beam of ultrasound in use for recording M-mode scan and traversing mitral valve. (B) shows 2DE sector scan covering section in long axis of the heart.

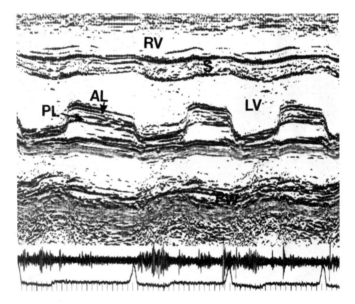

Fig. 1.11 Rheumatic mitral stenosis. The M-mode echocardiogram shows the characteristic features of this condition: the diastolic closure rate of the anterior mitral valve leaflet (AL) is reduced and the posterior leaflet (PL) moves forward in parallel with the anterior leaflet, due to commissural fibrosis which impedes leaflet separation. RV = right ventricle; LV = left ventricle.

duce the images in 'real time', i.e., unlike the static B-scan picture actual motion is shown as it occurs. The special probes used are complex linear, phased or sector scanners. Moving parts such as heart valves can be seen in motion, and the method is widely used in cardiology (two-dimensional echocardiography or 2DE) (Figs 1.10B and 1.12).

Doppler. The velocity of blood flow towards or away from an ultrasound probe can be derived from the reflected ultrasound wave using the well known Doppler principle. The effect has found widespread use in fetal monitoring, cardiology and vascular studies.

Duplex scanners combine both pulse echo ultrasound and Doppler shift facilities. Both modes can be simultaneously recorded.

Continuous wave Doppler uses two transducer crystals mounted side by side, one transmitting and the other receiving ultrasound waves. The method is best for measuring high velocity flow and for recording peak velocities.

Pulsed Doppler uses a single transducer to emit short bursts of ultrasound which are received back by the same transducer and

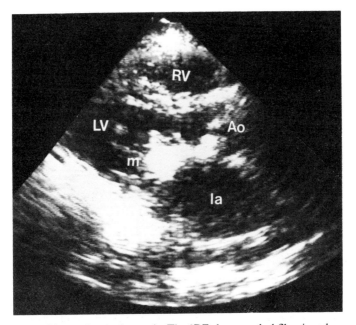

Fig. 1.12 Rheumatic mitral stenosis. The 2DE shows marked fibrosis and tethering of the mitral (m) leaflects due to chordal and commissural fusion. Ao = aorta; la = left artrium. Compare Fig 1.10B

recorded in the intervals between emission pulses. This method permits precise focussing on small sample volumes but is less accurate than continuous wave Doppler for peak and high velocity flow.

Colour flow mapping is based on pulsed Doppler but allows assessment across the whole field of a two dimensional image. The results can be coded in colour permitting immediate visual recognition of flow towards or away from the transducer.

MRI

Magnetic resonance imaging (MRI) represents the most exciting advance in imaging since medical radiology began in 1895. It has also been labelled nuclear magnetic resonance (NMR) and is based on the fact that some nuclei – those with unpaired electrons – behave like tiny magnets. Hydrogen nuclei (protons) are particularly suitable since they are normally present in vast numbers in the body tissues. Water for instance has 10^{23} per ml. The use of a strong external magnetic field will force a proportion of these nuclei to align in a new magnetic axis from their previous random orientation (Fig. 1.13). The fields used in clinical practice range from 0.15 to 1.5 Tesla (1500 to 15 000 Gauss) as compared with the earth's magnetic field of 0.5 Gauss.

In addition to the large and costly magnet required for MRI the machine also uses pulses of radiowaves. These are essential to excite and detect the magnetised protons. A pulse of radiowaves of the

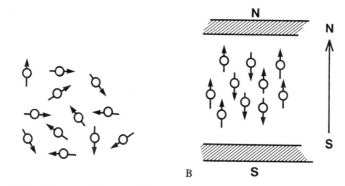

Fig. 1.13 Diagram to illustrate (A) random orientation of protons behaving like tiny bar magnets, (B) alignment of protons when immersed in a strong external magnetic field.

appropriate frequency displaces nuclei from their new alignment. They return to this immediately after the pulse ceases. At the same time they release the energy absorbed as a radiosignal of the same frequency. This is detected by the coils used for excitation (Fig. 1.14). Since the signal returned is proportional to the concentration of protons it forms the basis for a digital record of the proton content of the tissues under examination. Using a similar technique to that established in CT this is converted by computer into an analogue image presented on a cathode ray tube in varying shades of black and white.

In summary, the MR signal on which the image is based is produced by a radiofrequency (RF) pulse returned from RF stimulated protons in magnetised tissues.

The main RF pulse sequences used in MRI are labelled saturation recovery (SR), inversion recovery (IR) and spin echo (SE). The different pulse sequences give different weighting in the recovered signal to various parameters which affect the resulting image. Inversion recovery (T_1 weighted) sequences show better anatomical detail and better separation of solid and cystic structures. Spin echo (T_2 weighted) sequences are more sensitive to detecting local pathology.

Whilst MRI can produce axial images resembling those of CT it also has the great advantage that images can also be readily produced in any other plane including the sagittal and coronal, features of particular value in the study of the spine and brain. Other advantages compared with CT are the absence of ionising radiation or any other apparent biological hazard, and the high intrinsic contrast. The new method also holds out the promise of tissue characterisation and can be used for blood flow imaging.

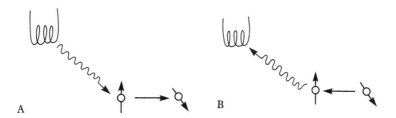

Fig. 1.14 Diagram to illustrate (A) effect of suitable radiofrequency pulse from external coil in displacing magnetised proton from its axis with absorption of energy. (B) Return of proton to its former axis with release of energy as radiofrequency pulse which can be registered by receiving coil and quantified.

Disadvantages of MRI are the high cost of the sophisticated machinery and inability to image bone and calcium. It is also unsuitable for patients with cardiac pacemakers which can be adversely affected by the magnetic fields as can metallic clips or implants.

2. The chest

The imaging investigations of the chest may be considered under the following headings:

1. Simple X-ray
2. Chest-screening
3. Tomography
4. Bronchography
5. Pulmonary angiography
6. Isotope scanning
7. Computed tomography
8. MRI
9. Needle biopsy.

Simple X-ray

In hospital practice many patients have a routine chest X-ray on admission. This is done not only to exclude serious chest disease, but also to provide evidence of the preoperative condition of the chest in patients about to undergo surgery. Postoperative chest complications include basal collapse, lung infections, and pulmonary embolus. In the assessment of such postoperative complications it is important to have a preoperative film for comparison. Chest X-ray also shows the size and shape of the heart and provides base line evidence of the cardiac status.

Simple radiography of the chest is also carried out as a routine in all patients with suspected chest disease. The study of chest X-rays requires an intimate knowledge of the normal anatomy of the lungs including the bronchi and their lobar and segmental arrangements (Fig. 2.1). Lesions must be anatomically localised and this will often require a lateral projection as well as a simple posteroanterior film. In studying the simple X-ray the radiologist will note not only the lung fields but also the heart and mediastinum, the pulmonary

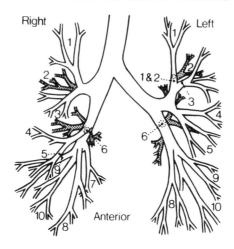

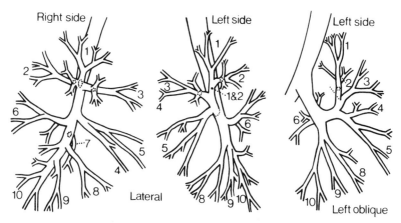

Fig. 2.1 Diagram illustrating the anatomy of the main bronchi and segmental divisions. Nomenclature approved by the Thoracic Society. (Reproduced by permission of the Editors of *Thorax*.)

UPPER LOBE
1. Apical bronchus
2. Posterior bronchus
3. Anterior bronchus

Right	*Left*
MIDDLE LOBE	LINGULA
4. Lateral bronchus	4. Superior bronchus
5. Medial bronchus	5. Inferior bronchus

LOWER LOBE

6. Apical bronchus	6. Apical bronchus
7. Medial basal (cardiac)	8. Anterior basal bronchus
8. Anterior basal bronchus	9. Lateral basal bronchus
9. Lateral basal bronchus	10. Posterior basal bronchus
10. Posterior basal bronchus	

vasculature, the position of the diaphragm, and the condition of the bony thorax.

Inspecting a chest X-ray

The student inspecting a chest film should try to examine it in a systematic manner. Though a radiologist may give an opinion, after what appears to the student only a cursory inspection, this is based on years of experience, and the examination of many thousands of films. The radiologist will have noted the normality or abnormality of all the following features:

1. The lung fields and pulmonary vessels
2. The heart and mediastinum
3. The diaphragm and subdiaphragmatic areas
4. The bony thorax (ribs, clavicles, scapulae, spine and shoulder joints)
5. The soft tissues (muscles, breast and cutaneous tissues).

The student should train himself to follow a routine which examines each of the above features in turn. In order to examine the lung fields and pulmonary vessels fully, it is helpful to divide each side of the chest into three zones – upper, middle and lower – and to check each in turn noting any deviation from the normal or difference from the other side. A similar systematic approach should be applied to the other features listed above, since significant abnormalities may be seen in any of them.

Thus an irregular bony defect in a rib with an adjacent soft tissue swelling may represent the first evidence of metastasis. An elevated diaphragm on one side with a small basal effusion may be evidence of a subphrenic abscess. A small bulge of the upper mediastinum may represent a tumour or an aneurysm. These few examples serve to illustrate the importance of the simple chest film in identifying disease not only of the lung parenchyma but also of many other systems.

Chest screening

In the early days of radiology chest screening was regarded as an essential part of the examination of the chest. Chest screening, however, involves an increased dose of irradiation to the patient compared with a simple chest X-ray. In practice it is now only carried out for the elucidation of specific problems. Thus it may be used to determine whether the diaphragm is moving normally or is paralysed; to assess the relationship of an opacity to other structures more accurately by observing it with different degrees of rotation on the screen; or to confirm valvar or other intracardiac calcification since this is much better visualised by screening with an image intensifier than on a simple film.

Tomography

This is used for the clearer demonstration of doubtful opacities in the lung field (Fig. 2.2); for the better visualisation of masses or

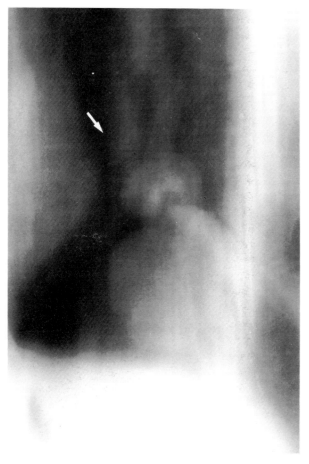

Fig. 2.2   Tomogram of basal pulmonary opacity confirms that it is due to an angioma. Note the tortuous dilated vein ($\rightarrow$).

apparent masses at the lung hila (Fig. 2.11); for the study of the margins of opacities in the lung – whether clear-cut or infiltrating surrounding lung; and for the better demonstration of cavities or suspected cavities within a lung lesion, or of calcification in an opacity.

Bronchography

This procedure is now little used and mainly for the demonstration of bronchiectasis (Fig. 2.3). It is also sometimes used for the

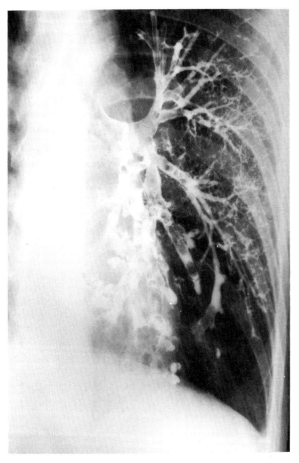

Fig. 2.3 Bronchogram showing good filling of the left bronchial tree. There is bronchiectasis involving the left lower lobe and part of the lingula.

demonstration of an obstructed or stenosed bronchus in suspected carcinoma.

Bronchography is performed in the X-ray department by the radiologist. There are several techniques available.

The contrast medium, propyliodine (Dionosil), can be injected over the back of the tongue, or through the nares, or directly through the cricothyroid membrane. In all cases the trachea is first rendered anaesthetic by means of local anaesthesia. Once the contrast medium has been injected the patient is tilted into the various positions necessary for filling the appropriate lobes of the lung with contrast (Fig. 2.3).

Pulmonary angiography

Pulmonary angiography is performed by passing a catheter from a peripheral vein through the right atrium and right ventricle into the main pulmonary artery and then if necessary into the right or left pulmonary artery. Contrast medium is injected so as to opacify the blood supply of the area under examination. The main use of the method is to confirm a suspected diagnosis of *pulmonary embolus.*

Pulmonary angiography is also occasionally used for the elucidation of opacities in the lung fields; e.g., to confirm a diagnosis of arteriovenous fistula or angiomatous malformation in the lung. Most of these cases, however, can be diagnosed by simple X-ray or tomography (Fig. 2.2).

Radioisotope scanning

Radioisotope scanning of the lungs is widely practised to confirm or refute a clinical diagnosis or suspicion of pulmonary embolus. If the findings are normal the more invasive pulmonary angiography can be dispensed with, and if they are abnormal and typical treatment may be instituted.

Lung scans can be performed following intravenous injection of technetium ($^{99}Tc^m$) labelled macroaggregates or microspheres. This is known as the perfusion or P scan. It can also be performed by inhalation of radioactive xenon (^{133}Xe) or krypton ($^{81}Kr^m$). This is known as the ventilation or Q scan.

If the perfusion scan is normal no further action is required, but if it shows perfusion defects suggestive of embolism then a ventilation scan can be done. Typically in pulmonary embolus the lung remains aerated and the ventilation scan remains normal, giving rise to the so called 'mismatching' of the P and Q scans. This mismatch is virtually diagnostic of pulmonary emboli (Fig. 2.4).

Tuberculosis

With most chest diseases radiology mirrors the gross pathology of the disease. Tuberculosis, though no longer the ubiquitous and sinister threat of past decades, is still a problem that must be borne in mind, particularly with immigrants from underdeveloped countries and in the immunosuppressed patient.

The primary form of tuberculous infection, which used to be seen almost exclusively in children, is now also being seen in older patients. The characteristic X-ray picture of a primary tuberculous

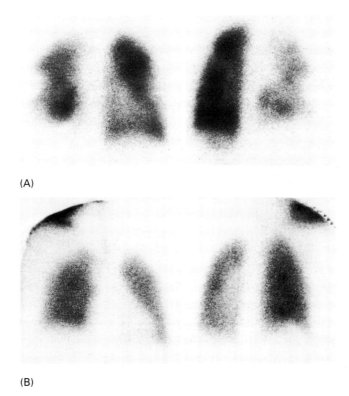

(A)

(B)

Fig. 2.4 (A) Perfusion lung scan with $^{99}Tc^m$ microspheres. There are several large defects in the right lung and a smaller defect in the left lung. (B) Same patient after ventilation scan with $^{87}Kr^m$. There are no ventilation defects. These mismatched perfusion and ventilation scans are characteristic of pulmonary embolus. AP views on Rt; PA views on L.

infection is an area of pneumonitis in the lung together with enlarged drainage glands at the affected hilum. This appears on the X-ray as a diffuse opacity representing a patch of consolidation in the lung field with increased striations extending towards the hilum where the enlarged glands show as rounded opacities. *Pleural effusion* is also a common manifestation of primary tuberculous infection.

The adult type of pulmonary tuberculosis (secondary or reactivated tuberculous infection) manifests in a different way. There is again an area of pneumonitis in the lung but this is not accompanied by glandular enlargement. The infection has a predilection for the posterior segment of the upper lobe. On the postero-anterior film it appears as an area of shadowing near the lung apex often mottled in character. Cavitation may occur, and as the disease progresses fibrosis will follow. The appearance in the majority of cases is characteristic both in the acute and chronic fibroid stages (Fig. 2.5).

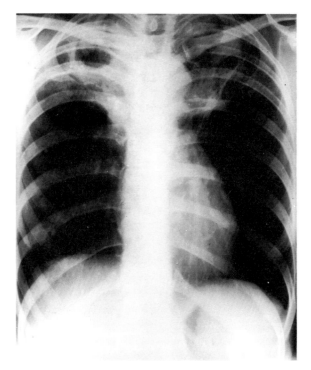

Fig. 2.5 Chronic fibroid tuberculosis of both upper lobes with cavitation.

Although the fulminating and serious forms of the disease are now rare in Britain they are by no means extinguished. Bronchogenic spread may occur from a tuberculous cavity, and on the X-ray this will appear as mottled small opacities in the newly invaded area. Miliary tuberculosis, being haematogenous, appears as fine pinpoint mottling spread uniformly throughout both lung fields.

With chronic fibroid tuberculosis in the upper lobes cavitation is quite common, but owing to the dense fibrous tissue tomography may be required for its demonstration.

Pneumonia and broncho-pneumonia

Pneumonia. With the widespread and early use of antibiotics for chest infections lobar pneumonia is less commonly seen than previously. In its classical form lobar pneumonia shows on the X-ray as an opacity outlining the whole anatomical distribution of a lobe (Fig. 2.6). As resolution occurs the dense opacity becomes irregular

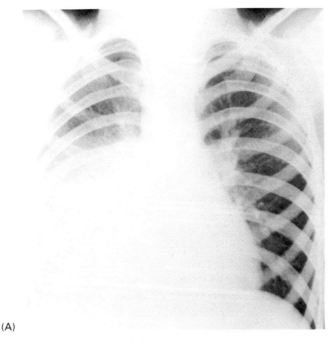

(A)

Fig. 2.6(A) Caption see overleaf.

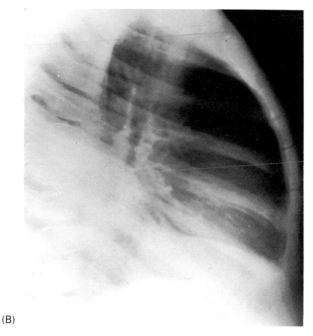

(B)

Fig. 2.6   Pneumonic consolidation of the right lower lobe: (A) postero-anterior film; (B) lateral film.

and mottled and the picture slowly improves to normality. With incomplete resolution fibrosis may occur and bronchiectasis may later supervene.

Legionnaires' disease occurs in sporadic or epidemic outbreaks due to *Legionella pneumophila* contaminating water coolers or air conditioning units. The chest X-ray shows a peripheral rapidly spreading consolidation. There is a 20% mortality.

Broncho-pneumonia is still commonly seen in hospital practice, particularly in elderly patients. The X-ray usually shows mottled shadowing, mainly in the lower lobes.

Local areas of *pneumonitis* are often seen in association with upper respiratory tract infection. These appear on the X-ray as an opacity localised to one segment of a lobe and resolving fairly rapidly.

The immunosuppressed patient (and the patient with AIDS) is particularly prone to lung infections, often with unusual pathogens. Certain organisms, notably *Pneumocystis carinii* and *cytomegalovirus* rarely if ever cause disease in the absence of immunosuppression.

Chronic bronchitis and emphysema

Although radiology is vital to the diagnosis of most chest conditions and in some cases will demonstrate lesions which cannot be shown by any other method, e.g. the small peripheral bronchial carcinoma, there is one field in which radiology may be entirely negative although the clinical evidence indicates serious chest disease. Thus a patient may have severe chronic bronchitis with gross physical signs on auscultation and severe clinical disability, yet X-rays may show little or nothing. This is because the bronchial walls are not normally visible on X-rays, and inflammation of the bronchial mucosa cannot be seen except by its secondary effects.

In severe cases there is usually some degree of *emphysema*. The latter is diagnosed at X-ray by the barrel-shaped deformity of the chest and by the flattened diaphragm. The lung fields may appear translucent and the hilar shadows prominent. In some cases of chronic bronchitis thickening of the bronchial walls due to peribronchial infection may occur and this may be seen on the X-ray. In severe cases of chronic bronchitis bronchography often shows characteristically enlarged mucous glands in the walls of the larger bronchi.

Bronchiectasis and lung abscess

Bronchiectasis may be suspected in the patient with recurrent infection, usually in the basal areas of the lung, or with the characteristic clinical picture of repeated infection and purulent foul-smelling sputum. In chronic cases there is usually increased shadowing in the affected area of the lung, sometimes with thickened bronchi visible on plain X-ray, or cystic shadows in the affected area. Bronchography was usually indicated to delineate the total extent of the disease since surgical removal of localised chronic bronchiectasis is the treatment of choice. Often bronchography will show that the disease is more extensive than is suggested in the plain X-rays (Fig. 2.3). Thin section CT now offers a non-invasive alternative to bronchography.

Lung abscess. Simple lung abscess is usually secondary to bronchial obstruction. This may be due to mucous plugs following a respiratory infection. The possibility of bronchial blockage by an inhaled foreign body should not be overlooked. The inhaled peanut is a notorious cause of bronchial occlusion with secondary infection in children. Most lung abscesses usually develop a fluid level visible on plain X-ray (Fig. 2.7).

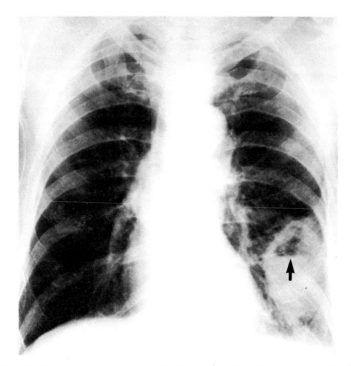

Fig. 2.7 Abscess cavity containing fluid level (↑). Note thin smooth wall and absence of any surrounding consolidation.

The pleura

Dry pleurisy is another condition in which clinical symptoms may be severe yet the radiological findings may be negative.

Pleural tumours are rare, but attention has been drawn to the frequency of malignant pleural tumours (*mesothelioma*) in asbestos workers. Linear pleural or diaphragmatic calcification is a frequent finding in asbestosis.

Pleural effusions manifest radiologically as basal peripheral opacities which first fill in the costophrenic angle (Fig. 2.8) and then extend up into the axilla. A large effusion may mask the whole of a lung field and even a moderate-sized effusion may obscure underlying lung disease. Pleural effusions were often a manifestation of primary tuberculous infection. They are now less often seen accompanying pneumonia or as post-pneumonic complications.

In the middle-aged or elderly person the possibility that a pleural effusion may be *malignant* must always be considered. As is well

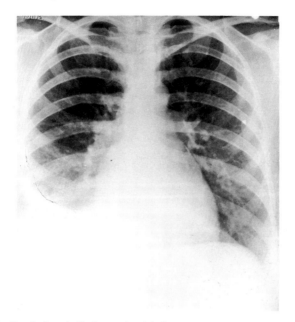

Fig. 2.8 Small pleural effusion at the right base.

known, malignant effusions may be bloodstained and will recur rapidly on tapping.

Apart from the inflammatory effusions and those associated with malignant disease, pleural effusions may also be seen as complications of heart failure, hepatic failure or the nephrotic syndrome.

Empyema, once a common post-pneumonic complication, is now rarely seen.

Spontaneous pneumothorax (Fig. 2.9) occurs usually in young patients and the etiology often remains obscure. In some cases rupture of an emphysematous bulla is inferred. In others there may be a subpleural tuberculous focus. In most cases, however, the etiology is never established. A small pneumothorax is usually better shown by obtaining a film taken in expiration as well as the routine inspiration film.

Traumatic pneumothorax is often seen in association with chest and rib injuries. *Tension pneumothorax* is a particularly dangerous condition when air continues to enter the pneumothorax but cannot escape owing to the pleural tear being valvular. It should be suspected if there is displacement of the mediastinum and over-distension of the affected side of the chest, and requires emergency treatment.

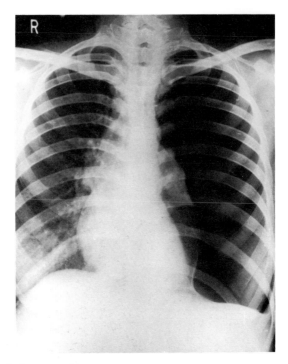

Fig. 2.9 Left pneumothorax.

The pneumoconioses

In this group of conditions foreign substances are inhaled and stored in the lungs. They are of considerable industrial importance and occur in many different occupations, including mining and industries using abrasives and refractories. Some of the inhaled foreign materials are capable of producing extensive fibrosis and a severe effect on lung function. These include silica, asbestos, talc, and beryllium.

Silicosis is due to the inhalation of small particles of silicon dioxide. In the advanced stages of the disease there is widespread nodulation and fibrosis throughout the lung fields and tuberculosis was a common complication. With modern industrial precautions the severe cases are now less commonly seen but it is important for the radiologist to recognise the early changes of pneumoconiosis. These may consist merely of a slight exaggeration of the normal lung markings. As the disease advances this increases to small nodules, a few millimetres in diameter, scattered throughout the lung fields (Fig. 2.10).

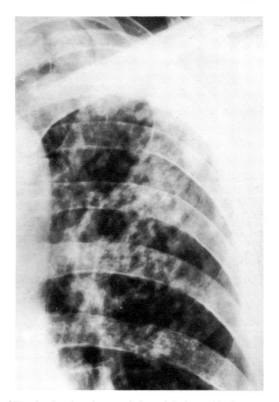

Fig. 2.10 Silicosis, showing characteristic nodulation, with clear cut outlines.

Sarcoidosis

Sarcoidosis is characterised by non-caseating granulomatous lesions which affect pulmonary, lymphatic, dermal and uveal tract tissues and occasionally bone. Enlargement of the mediastinal lymphatic glands is a frequent and early manifestation and may be the sole radiological lesion. The glands involved are bronchopulmonary and appear as bilateral symmetrical hilar and peri-hilar masses (Fig. 2.11).

The lesions slowly resolve over a period varying from six months to two years. Miliary lung mottling is also an early manifestation of sarcoidosis and may or may not accompany the hilar glandular enlargement. It usually disappears in a few months but may be followed by chronic pulmonary fibrosis. Large nodular lung lesions are unusual but are sometimes seen as a manifestation of pulmonary sarcoidosis, and these can persist for years.

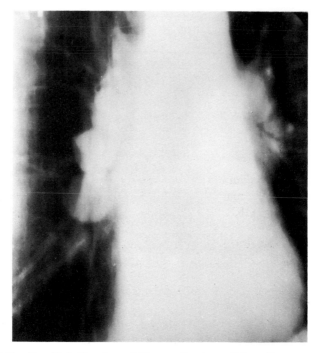

Fig. 2.11   *Sarcoidosis.* Female aged 33 years. Routine radiology discovery. Considered clinically to be sarcoidosis. Tomography demonstrates enlargement of the broncho-pulmonary (hilar) and tracheobronchial glands of both sides. The right hilar region shows the lobulation characteristic of enlarged lymph glands. Complete resolution within a year.

Tumours of mediastinum

Lymphoma

Hodgkin's disease is the most frequent type of lymphoma to affect the mediastinum. The paratracheal glands are the ones most frequently involved leading to enlargement and widening of the superior mediastinum. The *non-Hodgkin's lymphomas* can give rise to similar changes and *leukaemia* can also present similar radiological appearances.

Hodgkin's disease and the other lymphomas usually show a marked initial response to radiotherapy. This is in contrast to glands involved by bronchial carcinoma which sometimes have to be considered in differential diagnosis.

Other masses which enter into the radiological differential diagnosis on a PA chest film include the following:

Anterior mediastinal	Retrosternal thyroid
	Thymic tumour or cyst
	Aneurysm
	Terato-dermoid cyst
Middle mediastinal	Sarcoidosis
	Bronchogenic cyst
	Aortic aneurysm
Posterior mediastinal	Neuro-enteric cyst
	Neurogenic tumour
	Dilated oesophagus (achalasia)

A lateral chest film is of course essential to localise and help in elucidating the mass seen on the PA film. In difficult cases CT (Fig. 2.12) or MRI may prove invaluable in characterising a mediastinal mass.

MRI has the added attraction of distinguishing aneurysms and other vascular structures without injection of contrast (Fig. 2.13).

Lung tumour

Benign tumours of the lung are rare compared with malignant tumours. They include *bronchial adenoma* and *hamartomas*. The latter can sometimes be diagnosed on X-ray by the presence of irregular calcification within the tumour. This occurs in about 30% of these cases.

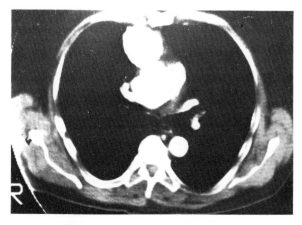

Fig. 2.12 Enhanced CT shows rounded mass anterior to the contrast opacified aorta and right pulmonary artery. Thymoma confirmed at surgery.

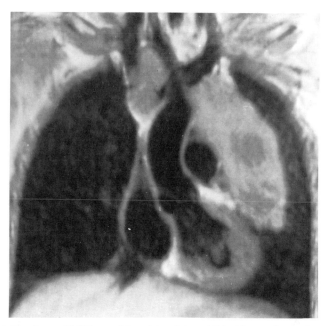

Fig. 2.13 Coronal MRI scan (T_1-weighted) in a child with a mediastinal mass. Note how the heart and great vessels are readily differentiated by low signal due to blood flow from the glandular masses due to Hodgkin's disease.

Bronchial carcinoma

Radiology plays an essential part in the early diagnosis and students should be aware of the protean radiological manifestations of the condition. The radiological appearances in bronchial carcinoma can be discussed under three main headings:

1. The visualisation of the primary tumour mass
2. Visualisation not of the tumour, but of its secondary effects or complications
3. Visualisation of glandular or other metastases from the primary lesion.

1. The primary tumour may be shown as a nodular opacity in the lung fields (Fig. 2.14). In a patient over 40 the possibility that any rounded lesion in the lung periphery may be a primary carcinoma must always be borne in mind. Nowadays the condition must even be considered in patients in their thirties or younger. In many of these cases it is quite impossible to exclude malignancy and needle biopsy must be undertaken. Solitary pulmonary nodules or

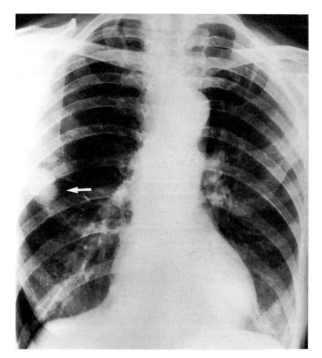

Fig. 2.14 Peripheral nodular carcinoma in the right mid-zone (◄).

Table 2.1 Causes of a solitary pulmonary nodule

Malignant tumours:	Primary, secondary, lymphoma, plasmacytoma
Benign tumours:	Hamartoma, adenoma, arteriovenous malformation
Granuloma:	Tuberculosis, histoplasmosis, paraffinoma, fungi, parasites
Infections:	Pneumonia, abscesses, hydatid, amoebic abscess
Pulmonary infarct	
Pulmonary haematoma	
Collagen diseases:	Rheumatoid arthritis, Wegener's granulomatosis
Sarcoidosis	
Sequestrated segment	
Retention cyst	
Impacted mucus	
Amyloid	
Intrapulmonary lymph node	
Pleural:	Fibroma, tumour, loculated fluid
Non-pulmonary	e.g. skin lesions

'coin lesions' are most commonly tumours, primary or secondary, or granulomata, but there are many other causes (Table 2.1).

The primary lesion may also be seen as an opacity at or near the hilum of the lung (Fig. 2.15). It is often difficult to be certain whether such an opacity represents the actual primary or a glandular metastasis. Fortunately, most of the hilar lesions are within reach of the bronchoscope and rapid confirmation of the diagnosis can usually be obtained.

2. A bronchial carcinoma will often occlude the bronchus in which it arises and this will lead to secondary collapse of the affected segment or lobe of the lung. Infection may then occur in the collapsed or partially collapsed area. X-rays may demonstrate these secondary effects without showing the original lesion. For this reason an unexplained area of collapse or consolidation in the lung fields in a man of carcinoma age must always be regarded with suspicion. An area of infection distal to a partially blocked bronchus may give rise to a difficult problem of differential diagnosis. Thus

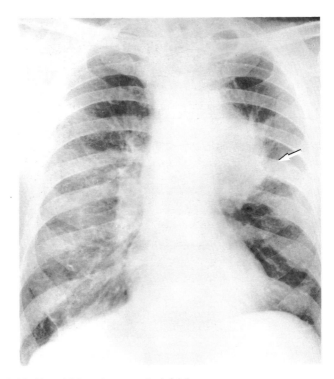

Fig. 2.15 Bronchial carcinoma at the left hilum.

a cavitating lung lesion may represent a simple lung abscess, a lung abscess distal to a bronchus obstructed by carcinoma, or a cavitating primary carcinoma.

3. As already noted, a hilar mass may represent not the primary tumour but *glandular metastases*. Peripheral lesions or metastases involving the pleura may result in *pleural effusion*. Characteristically the malignant effusion may be blood-stained and will recur rapidly after tapping. The pathologist may demonstrate malignant cells in the fluid. A hilar carcinoma or glandular metastases may involve the phrenic nerve. This will manifest itself by elevation of the diaphragm on the affected side, and on screening the affected dome will be seen to move paradoxically.

With an apical (or Pancoast) tumour there is often direct invasion of ribs, with bony destruction apparent on X-rays (Fig. 2.16). Bony metastases may occur elsewhere in the body and will manifest themselves as destructive areas on X-ray or by pathological fractures.

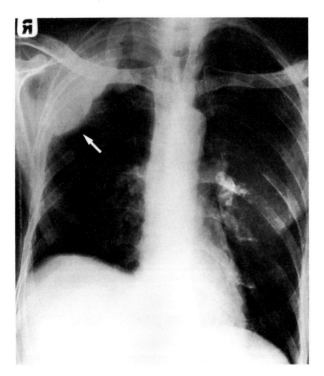

Fig. 2.16 Tumour at the right apex eroding ribs. Note the high diaphragm due to phrenic paralysis.

Once the diagnosis of carcinoma of the lung has been made or confirmed, radiology is also useful in assessing operability. Evidence of metastases usually precludes operation. By demonstrating large glands encroaching on the oesophagus a barium swallow may save a useless thoracotomy. If involvement of the superior vena cava is suspected this should be conformed by superior vena cavography or CT and again a useless thoracotomy may be prevented.

Secondary deposits

The lungs are a common site for the development of metastases. Haematogenous tumour emboli are carried to the heart and then become lodged in the capillaries of the pulmonary circulation. Thus X-ray of the lungs is necessary in most forms of malignant disease. Secondary deposits in the lungs usually appear as rounded opacities which can be multiple and widespread (Fig. 2.17). Large so-called 'cannon-ball' secondary deposits may be seen with certain types of

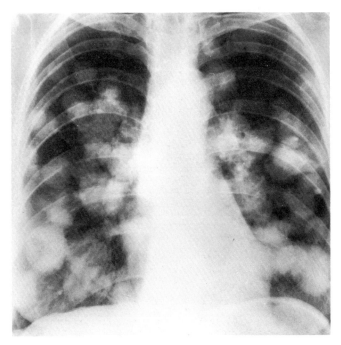

Fig. 2.17   Discrete metastases. Carcinoma of breast. The lung between lesions is normal.

primary tumour: e.g. osteogenic sarcoma, seminoma of the testis and hypernephroma. Secondary deposits can also present a variety of different appearances, ranging from miliary mottling throughout the lung fields to extensive perihilar spread (lymphangitis carcinomatosa).

Needle biopsy

Peripheral tumours in the lung which are normally beyond the reach of bronchoscopic investigation are now biopsied percutaneously by the radiologist using a fine needle. Under image intensifier control the tip of the needle is advanced to the lesion and a biopsy obtained by suction as the needle is passed into the lesion. Occasional complications of the procedure are pneumothorax and haematemesis but these usually require no treatment and are preferable to the alternative of thoracotomy.

Ultrasound

Ultrasound is helpful in assessing pleural and subphrenic disease and is invaluable in cardiac lesions (see Ch. 3). It has however no significant part to play in the diagnosis of pulmonary lesions.

CT

The main use of CT in the chest is in assessing mediastinal disease and in staging of lung cancer and other malignant lesions. It is also more sensitive than simple X-ray in identifying small pulmonary metastases and in detecting pulmonary fibrosis and bronchiectasis. High resolution thin section CT (HRCT) is invaluable in elucidating interstitial pulmonary disease.

MRI

MRI of the chest has proved most valuable in the assessment and characterisation of mediastinal masses (Fig. 2.13). Its ability to show sections in the sagittal and coronal as well as the axial plane and its ability to show vascular structures without contrast injections give it an advantage over CT. It is also useful in the diagnosis of hilar and mediastinal lymphadenopathy and in the staging of malignant tumours.

3. The heart

Imaging of the heart will be considered under the following headings:

1. Simple X-ray
2. Screening
3. Cardiac catheterisation
4. Angiocardiography
5. Coronary arteriography
6. Ultrasound
7. Isotope scanning
8. MRI.

Simple X-rays

A simple X-ray of the chest is mandatory as the first imaging investigation in cases of heart disease, because it yields vital information concerning the size of the heart, enlargement of individual chambers and condition of the lung fields. All these features are important in the assessment of the nature of the specific heart disease and its severity. An initial chest X-ray also forms a base line against which future progress or deterioration can be measured.

Size of heart. This is measured by the cardio-thoracic (CT) ratio. The maximum transverse diameter (TD) of the heart is compared with the maximum transverse diameter of the thorax (Fig. 3.1). In normal adults this is less than 50% in a film taken at the standard 6 foot (tube to film) distance.

Shape of heart. The cardiac contour has characteristic appearances in specific conditions depending on the chambers mainly enlarged. *Left ventricular enlargement* is seen in hypertension, aortic valve disease and other conditions where the main burden is on the left ventricle. It manifests by enlargement of the apical region of the heart in both the PA and lateral projections (Figs 3.2A and 3.3).

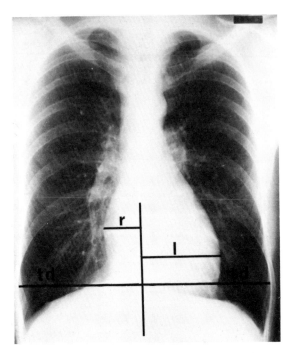

Fig. 3.1 The assessment of cardiac enlargement. The cardiac diameter should be the maximum cardiac diameter (r + 1). The transverse thoracic diameter is measured in a variety of ways. Here it is measured as the maximum internal diameter of the thorax.

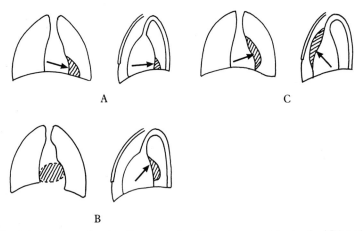

Fig. 3.2 Diagram showing directions of cardiac enlargement in standard PA and lateral views in (A) left ventricular, (B) left auricular and (C) right ventricular enlargement.

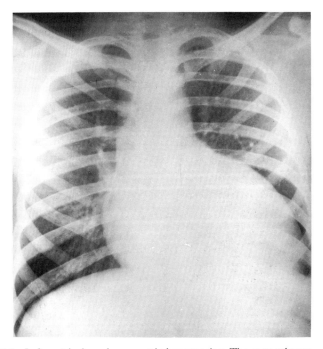

Fig. 3.3 Left ventricular enlargement in hypertension. The apex enlarges downwards and to the left.

Left auricular enlargement is seen characteristically in mitral valve disease, when it enlarges backwards and to the right, appearing as an added density superimposed on the central part of the heart shadow in the PA view. It projects backwards and slightly upwards in the lateral view, presenting a marked impression on the barium filled oesophagus (Figs 3.2B and 3.4). *Right ventricular enlargement* may also be seen in mitral disease because of the increased pulmonary resistance secondary to the pulmonary congestion. It is also seen in many congenital cardiac lesions associated with pulmonary stenosis or left to right shunts, and in pulmonary conditions with chronic airways obstruction. The enlarged right ventricle is best seen in the lateral view where it fills in the normal retrosternal space, but is also identifiable when gross in the PA view where it straightens the left border and elevates the apex of the heart (Fig. 3.2C). In mitral disease the combination of left auricular and right ventricular enlargement leads to the 'cottage loaf' appearance (Fig. 3.5).

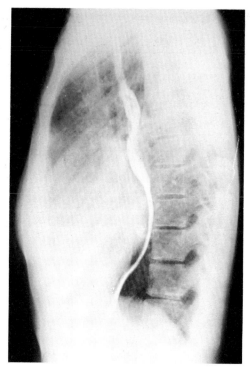

Fig. 3.4   Backward displacement of barium filled oesophagus by enlarged left auricle.

The lung fields

The appearance of the lung fields is of great importance in cardiac assessment since alterations in pulmonary haemodynamics are a feature of many forms of heart disease. Three types of change can be identified:

1. *Congestion.* This is due to *pulmonary venous hypertension,* which follows left heart lesions, resulting in back pressure on the lungs. Left ventricular failure or mitral disease are typical causes. The characteristic features are diversion of blood from the lower to the upper zones of the lung in the erect PA film. Normally the upper zone vessels appear smaller than those in the lower zone, but with pulmonary venous hypertension they become more prominent. As pressure rises pulmonary oedema develops involving the interstitial or alveolar spaces or both. Most characteristic are *septal lines* at the costo-phrenic angles representing fluid in the interlobular

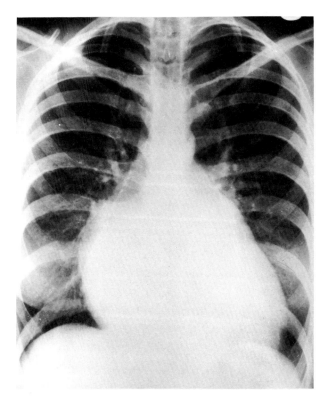

Fig. 3.5 Mitral stenosis. Note enlargement of the pulmonary conus and small aortic knuckle. The enlarged left auricle in this case projects as a rounded opacity to the right as well as backwards.

tissue planes (Fig. 3.6), and lamellar effusions in the parietal sub-pleural spaces or in the fissures. *Alveolar oedema* is often peri-hilar with blurring and haziness of the central lung areas ('bat's wing shadows'), but may be more widespread (Fig. 3.7). *Pleural effusions* may also develop, most commonly on the right, and may loculate, particularly in the fissures.

2. *Pulmonary plethora.* This is seen in conditions of high pul-monary flow mainly due to *congenital left to right heart shunts* and the degree of plethora roughly parallels flow provided pulmonary arterial pressure remains normal. Both arteries and veins become more prominent, particularly the arteries, with end on vessels close to the hilum being particularly well seen and distal vessels extend-ing out to the lung periphery. Extreme pulmonary arterial hyper-tension may complicate any shunt whether at atrial, ventricular

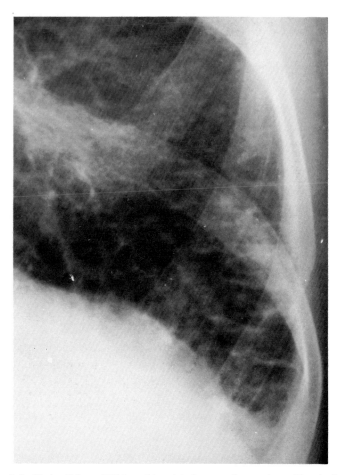

Fig. 3.6 Kerley B lines. Thickened interlobular septa in a patient with mitral valve disease seen as horizontal lines in the CP angle (septal lines).

or aortopulmonary level (Eisenmenger syndrome), with the shunt then becoming right to left. Major degrees of pulmonary plethora with giant central arteries are seen where the shunt is of long standing before hypertension develops, as in some cases of ASD where patients may reach the twenties before this occurs.

Pulmonary arterial hypertension (PAH) may also arise from the increased resistance produced by severe pulmonary venous hypertension, or from so-called primary PAH. It may also arise acutely from massive pulmonary embolus or from chronic multiple small pulmonary emboli. Finally it may be seen in chronic pulmonary disease with chronic airways obstruction.

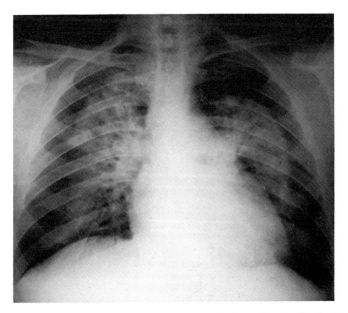

Fig. 3.7 Acute intra-alveolar pulmonary oedema with a bat's wing distribution around the hila.

3. *Pulmonary oligaemia* is seen when there is obstruction to the pulmonary outflow at or below the pulmonary valves, especially with a right to left shunt as in Fallot's tetralogy (Fig. 3.11).

Pericardial effusion

Pericardial effusions may be classified as:

1. *Inflammatory*
   a. Tuberculous
   b. Rheumatic
   c. Suppurative
   d. Viral
2. *Non-inflammatory*
   a. Heart failure
   b. Uraemia
   c. Myocardial infarction
   d. Haemopericardium
      i. Traumatic
      ii. Post-cardiac or aortic rupture
3. *Malignant.*

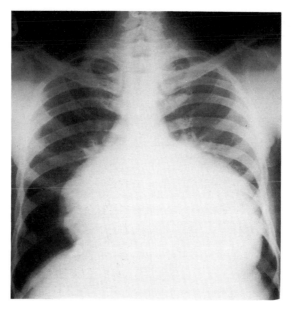

Fig. 3.8 Massive pericardial effusion enlarging heart and masking both hila.

The radiological diagnosis can be difficult unless the amount of fluid exceeds 200 ml. However, above this amount the appearances are fairly typical. The heart becomes globular with masking of the hila (Fig. 3.8). In doubtful cases the diagnosis can be confirmed by ultrasound. CT or MRI will also readily show small effusions.

Constrictive pericarditis may follow viral or tuberculous pericarditis and is occasionally seen following collagen diseases and haemopericardium. There is thickening and rigidity of the pericardium leading to constriction and impaired filling of the heart. The right heart is mainly involved leading to the clinical features of right heart failure. The heart may appear normal in size, but pericardial calcification, best seen in lateral view, is present in 50% of cases (Fig. 3.9).

Screening

Cardiac calcification is better seen at screening with an image intensifier than on a simple film. Calcification is most commonly seen in the mitral or aortic valves, but may also be seen in atheromatous coronary arteries, in the mitral annulus, or in a left atrium containing mural thrombus.

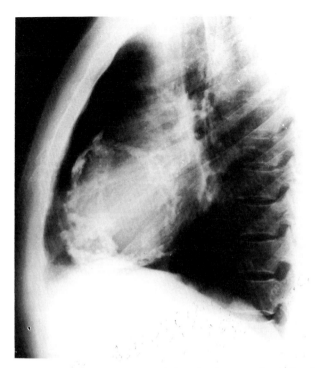

Fig. 3.9 Constrictive pericarditis. Lateral view showing extensive pericardial calcification spreading over the front of the right ventricle and also encircling the heart in the atrio-ventricular groove. There is no calcium at the back as fluid cannot collect there.

Screening the heart is essential for cardiac catheterisation, angiocardiography, left ventriculography, and coronary arteriography.

Cardiac catheterisation

This procedure requires the introduction of a catheter into the heart and manipulation of its tip under screen control so as to enter different chambers of the heart or to pass through abnormal defects or communications.

Right heart catheterisation. This can be performed percutaneously or after surgical exposure of a vein in the arm or groin, and passage of a catheter from there to the right atrium. The tip is manipulated into the right ventricle or beyond into the pulmonary artery or lung fields (Figs 3.10 and 3.11). If there is an atrial septal defect, ventricular septal defect, or patent ductus present, the catheter

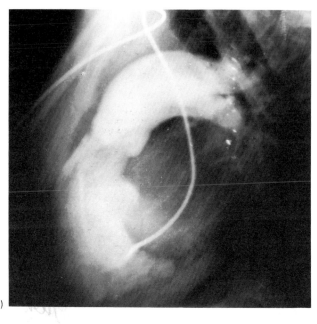

(A)

(B)

Fig. 3.10 Selective angiocardiograms. (A) The catheter tip is sited in the right ventricular outflow tract, just below the pulmonary valves (lateral view). (B) The catheter tip is sited in the main pulmonary artery (lateral view).

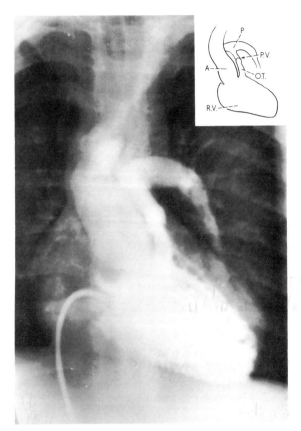

Fig. 3.11 Right ventricular angiogram of Fallot's tetralogy (AP view) showing hypoplastic RV outflow tract and deformed small pulmonary valve.
Diagram: A = aorta; P = pulmonary artery; RV = right ventricle; PV = pulmonary valve; OT = outflow tract.

may be passed to the left atrium, left ventricle or aorta through the defect. The site of the catheter tip can be confirmed by taking pressure recordings during the investigation and also by taking blood samples which are examined for oxygen saturation. The pressure recordings and oxygen saturation levels are of vital importance in the diagnosis of the different forms of congenital heart disease.

In many cases simple cardiac catheterisation, by obtaining intracardiac pressures and oxygen saturations in the affected cardiac chambers, is sufficient for precise diagnosis. In other cases, angiocardiography was also performed to obtain an accurate anatomical diagnosis.

Left heart catheterisation. The usual technique of left heart catheterisation is for the radiologist to introduce a catheter percutaneously into the femoral artery and to pass it under screen control into the aortic arch and through the aortic valves into the left ventricle. Pressures are obtained from inside the ventricle and recorded, as is a withdrawal pressure trace into the aorta.

Angiocardiography

Angiocardiography may be performed from either the right or the left side of the heart. In *venous angiocardiography* the catheter tip was sited either in the superior or inferior vena cava, and a bolus of contrast medium injected at high pressure. Rapid films were taken demonstrating its passage through the various chambers of the heart.

Right heart angiocardiography is now more usually performed by siting the catheter tip in the right atrium. In many congenital heart conditions *selective angiocardiography* is performed with the catheter tip sited in the right ventricle or pulmonary outflow tract (Figs 3.10 and 3.11). The left side of the heart can also be shown by following the contrast through the lungs to the left auricle and ventricle on serial films. However contrast values are not so good as in direct left heart ventriculography.

For *left heart angiocardiography* the catheter tip is sited in the left ventricle by the method of transfemoral catheterisation just described. Injections are made through the catheter and rapid serial films taken. The left ventricle is best studied by cine-filming, and this method is essential in the study of the ischaemic heart in coronary disease. Left ventricular function is assessed radiologically by noting the adequacy of left ventricular contraction and the presence of areas of dyskinesia. Mitral incompetence can be demonstrated at left ventriculography by opacification of the left auricle and the degree of incompetence quantified.

The aortic valves may be studied by injections made into the root of the aorta. With aortic incompetence there will be regurgitation into the left ventricle; with aortic stenosis the narrowed jet of blood from the ventricle will be shown as a defect in the opacified aorta.

Coronary arteriography

Coronary arteriography involves direct injection of the coronary arteries. Specially shaped catheters are introduced percutaneously from the femoral artery and passed into the coronary ostia. Contrast medium is injected and cine-films obtained. With modern apparatus it is possible to obtain excellent quality angiograms demonstrating stenotic or other lesions of the coronary vessels (Fig. 3.12). This is essential if surgery is being considered in patients with ischaemic cardiac symptoms. Arteriography can also be used to assess the results of coronary surgery.

It is also possible to dilate an atheromatous stenosis during coronary arteriography using specially designed catheters with attached dilatable balloons (Gruntzig).

Echocardiography

Ultrasound has developed into one of the most important techniques for cardiac diagnosis. The basic principles are described in Chapter 1.

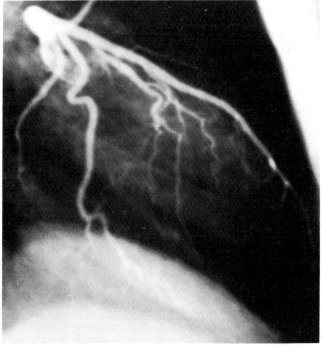

(A)

Fig. 3.12(A) Caption see overleaf.

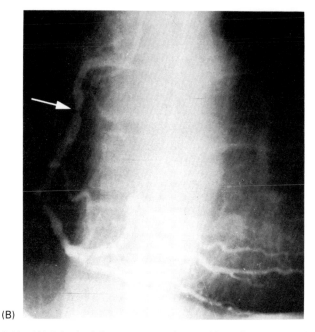

(B)

Fig. 3.12   (A) Selective left coronary arteriogram. Normal appearances in AP view. (B) Selective right coronary arteriogram. AP view shows stenosis of main right coronary artery (arrow).

M-mode (Figs 1.10, 1.11), once widely used, has now been supplanted by *two dimensional echocardiography* (2DE) (Figs 1.10, 1.12) which is also referred to as *cross sectional echocardiography* (CSE).

2DE uses a sector scanner and by making the ultrasound beam oscillate very rapidly backwards and forwards through an arc of 80° the information from a large number of M scans is combined to produce an accurate moving image of the section scanned. A moving real time image is thus obtained of the different sections or sectors of the heart being scanned.

Figure 3.13 illustrates diagrammatically the standard 'long axis' and 'short axis' views used. The 2DE provides definitive information on intracardiac anatomy in most neonates and children with congenital heart lesions (Fig. 3.14). It also provides definitive information in over 70% of adults with acquired heart lesions (Fig. 1.12). The limiting factor in other adults is the rib cage obstructing ultrasound access. In such cases the more invasive trans-oesophageal echocardiogram may be indicated (see below).

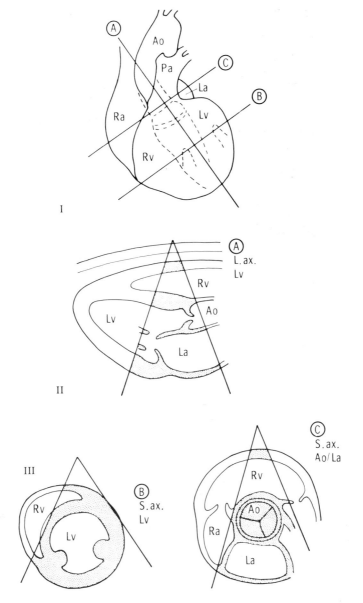

Fig. 3.13 CSE scanning of the heart. I The heart shown diagrammatically with the standard scanning planes indicated. (A) The long-axis view. (B) Short-axis view through the cavity of the left ventricle below the level of the mitral valve. (C) Short-axis view more cranially than in (B). Ao = aorta, La = left atrium, Lv = left ventricle, Lax = long-axis view, Pa = pulmonary artery, Ra = right atrium, Rv = right ventricle, Sax = short-axis view. II Long-axis view. III Short-axis views.

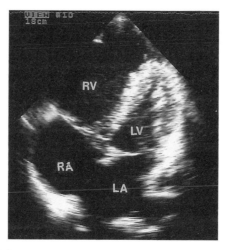

Fig. 3.14 Modified apical four-chamber echocardiogram of a patient with a secundum atrial septal defect. The right-sided chambers are considerably enlarged. LA = left atrium, RA = right atrium, LV = left ventricle, RV = right ventricle.

Doppler principles in the form of pulsed and continuous wave Doppler are used to obtain flow profiles of direction and average velocity of flow and thus show physiological aspects of intracardiac shunts and valvular disease. This information is obtained from a small area of interest and does not show flow images. *Colour flow mapping* (CFM) gathers Doppler shift information from multiple sample volumes along each CSE scan line. These are colour coded electronically to produce a display of flow direction and velocity. This will provide physiological information on areas of abnormal flow associated with intracardiac shunts or leaking or stenosed valves.

Transoesophageal echocardiography (TEE). This technique requires passage of an oesophagoscope with an ultrasound transducer at its tip which can be angled and placed at different levels behind the heart. This enables high quality CSE or CFM images to be obtained in cases where the conventional techniques are difficult or unsuccessful.

Radionuclide scanning

There are two main forms of cardiac scanning with radionuclides:

1. Myocardial imaging
2. Nuclear angiography.

Myocardial imaging can be achieved in two ways. Infarct scanning uses an isotope (^{99}Tc^m pyrophosphate) which accumulates in damaged myocardium, whilst perfusion scanning uses several isotopes, the most popular being thallium 201, which accumulates in normal but not in damaged or ischaemic myocardium (Fig. 3.15).

The main clinical indication for infarct scanning is to assess patients with inconclusive or equivocal evidence of a recent myocardial infarct. It is also used for prognostic purposes as there is some correlation between the size of the infarct abnormality and long term prognosis.

Nuclear angiography can also be done in two different ways.

1. *First pass technique* involves rapid i.v. injection of a bolus of a simple radionuclide (^{99}Tc^m pertechnetate). Its passage through the cardiac chambers is then recorded. The method is most useful for the study of intracardiac shunts.

2. *Multigated equilibrium studies* (MUGA) follow injection of an isotope which remains fixed within the vascular space (^{99}Tc^m labelled human serum albumen or red blood cells) thus labelling the total blood pool. Cardiac movement is then assessed by linking the recorder to ECG gating over several hundred cardiac cycles, the data being accumulated into one totalised cycle. The images can then be transferred to a continuous loop of cine film for viewing in cine mode.

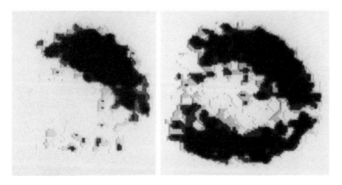

Fig. 3.15 Myocardial ischaemia. ^{201}Thallium citrate. Left: anterior image after exercise showing a large inferior defect. Right: 3 hours later, at equilibrium. Normal image. Thus there is exercise-induced transient myocardial ischaemia.

Abnormalities of ventricular function, particularly those due to ischaemic heart disease and cardiomyopathy are readily assessed by this method. Computer manipulation of the data also enables ventricular ejection fractions to be obtained.

Computed tomography

CT provides an excellent method of showing cardiac anatomy in the axial plane together with the great vessels and adjacent mediastinal structures. However intravenous contrast enhancement is usually necessary for most diagnostic purposes. This permits chamber identification and will show such features as intraventricular thrombus or the neck of a cardiac aneurysm (Fig. 3.16). Patency of coronary artery bypass grafts can also be shown by this technique.

MRI

Cardiac MRI is now well established and its use is expanding rapidly. The technique can provide information on both morphology and function. Its main attractions include high contrast between flowing blood and myocardium without the need for contrast medium or invasive techniques or radiation. It also readily

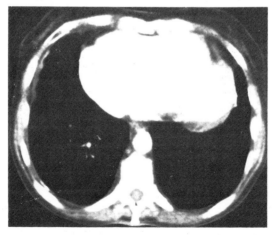

Fig. 3.16 Left ventricular aneurysm. Contrast enhancement demonstrates neck of apical and posterior aneurysm communicating with left ventricular cavity.

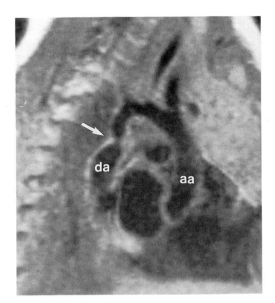

Fig. 3.17 Oblique sagittal gated spin-echo MR image in a child with coarctation of the aorta (arrowed). aa = ascending aorta, da = descending aorta. (Courtesy of the Trustees of the Bristol MRI Centre.)

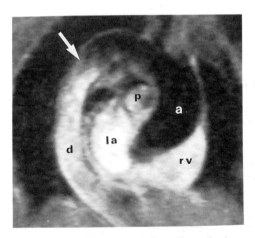

Fig. 3.18 Aortic stenosis on an oblique gated, gradient echo image (TE 22 ms) through the aortic arch during peak systole. Note signal loss, with a maximum measured length of 16 cm, extending to the descending aorta (arrowed), due to turbulent flow distal to the stenosed aortic valve (on cardiac catheterization the pressure gradient across the valve was 80 mmHG). a = ascending aorta, d = descending aorta, la = left atrium, p = pulmonary artery, rv = right ventricle.

provides multiplanar images including axial, coronal, sagittal and oblique views. As with CT the great vessels and adjacent mediastinal structures are also well shown. Images of the whole thoracic aorta can be easily obtained.

With modern techniques blood flow patterns can now be recognised and it may soon be possible to quantify stenotic and

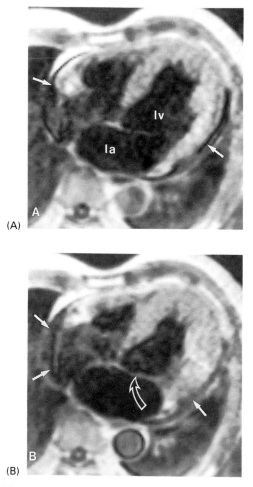

(A)

(B)

Fig. 3.19 Hypertrophic cardiomyopathy on transverse gated spin-echo images (TE 40 ms). (A) End-diastole. (B) End-systole. The myocardium is markedly thickened, with an associated pericardial effusion (straight arrows). la = left atrium, lv = left ventricle. (Adapted with permission from Jenkins & Isherwood 1987.)

regurgitant lesions as well as volume flow for cardiac output shunts etc.

Various cardiac lesions identified by MRI are illustrated in Figures 3.17, 3.18 and 3.19.

Ultrasound is of course cheaper and more easily available than MRI and is also radiation free and non invasive. It remains therefore the primary investigation of choice in most cardiac cases. MRI however is invaluable in cases where ultrasound fails or gives equivocal results.

4. The vascular system

The radiological investigation of the vascular system will be considered under the three headings of arteries, veins, and lymphatics.

Arteries

Several imaging methods can show the arteries in more or less detail, but *direct arteriography* is the technique most widely practised. Two basic methods are used:

1. Percutaneous needle puncture
2. Percutaneous arterial catheterisation.

The latter procedure is carried out using an ingenious instrument designed by Seldinger in Sweden. The technique is as follows:

The artery is punctured with a needle and a fine malleable guide wire is passed down the needle and into the lumen of the artery. The needle is withdrawn back over the guide and a catheter is then passed along the guide and through the puncture hole into the artery. The guide is then extracted through the catheter leaving the catheter in the artery. The latter can then be pushed along so that its tip lies at any level desired (Fig. 4.1).

The opaque catheters are screened by an image intensifier to confirm the correct level. The tips of these catheters can also be pre-shaped so as to enter branches of the aorta such as the renal arteries and provide a *selective arteriogram*.

These two techniques enable investigation of the whole of the arterial vascular tree to be undertaken in the X-ray department including selective angiography of such internal organs as kidney, liver, pancreas, spleen, brain, and heart.

The lower limb may be examined by needle puncture of the femoral artery in the groin, and the upper limb by catheterisation of the axillary or subclavian arteries from the femoral artery. The head

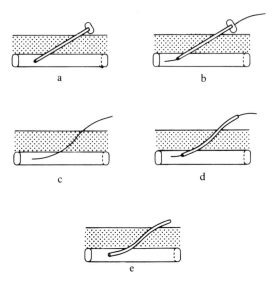

Fig. 4.1 Diagram to illustrate technique of percutaneous catheter insertion.
a. Needle inserted into artery.
b. Guide passed through needle into artery.
c. Needle withdrawn leaving guide in artery.
d. Catheter passed over guide into artery.
e. Guide withdrawn leaving catheter in artery.

and neck were originally examined by needle puncture of the common carotid or vetebral arteries in the neck, but catheter techniques from the femoral artery are now preferred. The abdominal aorta may be investigated by needle puncture of the aorta through the back (*lumbar aortography*). Alternatively, it can be investigated by percutaneous transfemoral catheterisation using the Seldinger technique. The thoracic aorta is examined by transfemoral catheterisation and passage of a catheter into the aortic arch (*arch aortography*). Where the femoral or iliac arteries are too diseased for this to be possible transaxillary catheterisation can be used.

Digital subtraction angiography (DSA) has been mentioned in Chapter 1. Computers are used to process digitalised information of the contrast bolus passing through the vessels of the target organ. The information is obtained from an intensifier screened image. The computer is able to subtract out the bones and other structures leaving only the opacified blood vessels on the analogue images obtained. The method is sensitive enough to obtain good arterial images from an intravenous bolus injection followed through the heart to the systemic circulation (Fig. 4.2). Arterial injections can

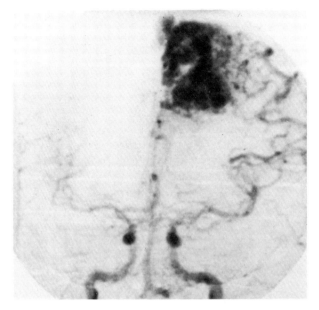

Fig. 4.2 Parasagittal angioma of the brain shown by intravenous DSA. AP view of the skull with bones subtracted. Both carotids and their branches are shown with the basilar artery centrally below the anterior cerebrals.

also be made using smaller and safer doses of contrast medium than with conventional arteriography.

Indications

The main clinical uses of arteriography can be considered under three headings:

1. Investigation of vascular disease
2. The diagnosis and differential diagnosis of tumours and cysts
3. Therapy (interventional angiography).

Vascular lesions

Atheromatous stenosis and thrombosis. This forms the largest group of cases seen in clinical practice. In the lower limb the *femoral artery* is a common site for these lesions and the patient presents with a characteristic history of intermittent claudication. With *iliac* lesions the picture is similar but the claudication affects the thigh muscles as well as the calf. Atheromatous stenosis and thrombosis may also occur in the *abdominal aorta* (Leriche syndrome, Fig. 4.3) and give rise to bilateral claudication which may affect the thigh and buttocks. With iliac or aortic thrombosis the appropriate femoral pulses will be absent.

Atheromatous stenosis and thrombosis is less common as a cause of disability in the upper limb but it is occasionally seen. It is also quite frequent at the origin of the *internal carotid artery* where it is known to be a common cause of remittent attacks of hemiplegia. Attention has also been drawn to atheromatous lesions in the *vertebral* arteries and in the intrathoracic *great vessels* as a cause of vertebro-basilar insufficiency.

Atheroma may involve the origin of the *renal artery* and lead to renal ischaemia with secondary hypertension. Arteriography has also demonstrated other causes of renal artery stenosis such as *fibromuscular hyperplasia* (Fig. 10.8, p. 177). This is a congenital developmental anomaly of the muscle wall of the artery leading to irregular beading and stenoses, and occurs mainly in young females.

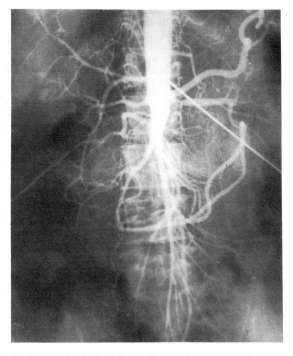

Fig. 4.3 Aortic thrombosis (Leriche syndrome) demonstrated by lumbar aortography.

Atheromatous stenosis of the *coronary arteries* may be associated with angina pectoris and cardiac ischaemia. Coronary arteriography is now widely practised and the surgical treatment of such lesions is now commonplace (see Ch. 3).

Embolism. This most commonly occurs in patients with atrial fibrillation and arises from atrial clot. Occasionally, cases are seen due to post-infarction clot in the left ventricle, or to paradoxical embolus. Arteriography will usually demonstrate the site and extent of the embolic lesion and may be helpful in deciding for or against surgical treatment (Fig. 4.4).

Aneurysms. Most of the aneurysms now seen in clinical practice are *degenerative* in origin and due to atheroma. In our experience the common sites have been the abdominal aorta and the popliteal artery (Fig. 4.5). As with atheroma generally there is a predominantly male sex incidence.

Infective aneurysms are less commonly seen and *syphilitic aneurysms* are becoming rare in this country. Most cases of syphilitic aneurysm are seen in the thoracic aorta. *Mycotic aneurysms* are also

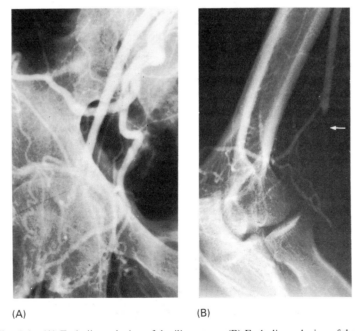

(A)　　　　　　　　　(B)

Fig. 4.4 (A) Embolic occlusion of the iliac artery. (B) Embolic occlusion of the brachial artery.

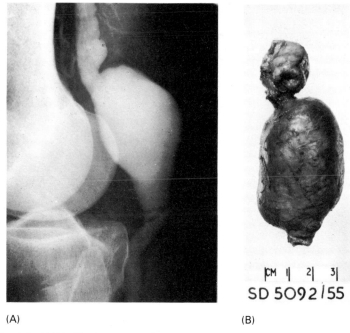

(A)   (B)

Fig. 4.5   (A) Popliteal aneurysm shown by arteriography. (B) Excised specimen.

relatively rare, but such aneurysms can enlarge very rapidly. *Traumatic aneurysms* are becoming increasingly common in this industrial and motor-car age (Fig. 4.6).

Dissecting aneurysms are now realised to be less uniformly fatal than was once thought. Surgery is now practised for the relief of some dissecting aneurysms and arteriography may be helpful to delineate the extent of the dissection (Fig. 4.7) though CT (and MRI if available) can now show the lesion non-invasively.

All the various types of aneurysm are well demonstrated by arteriography.

Arteriovenous fistula. A direct communication between an artery and a vein is usually traumatic and we are seeing an increasing number of cases. Occasional cases have followed surgery and we have seen several examples following orthopaedic operations on joints. Once an arteriovenous fistula has formed, the veins round the area become engorged with arterial blood, and the site of the fistula may be completely obscured at surgery. Arteriography is thus extremely helpful in localising the fistula, and making possible a successful surgical cure.

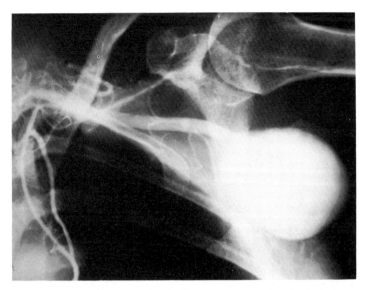

Fig. 4.6 Traumatic aneurysm of the axillary artery, shown by selective left subclavian catheterisation.

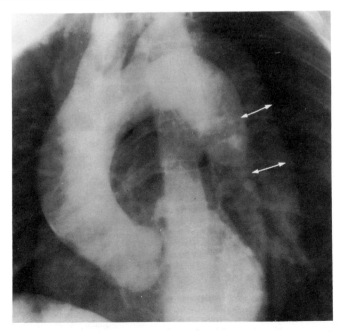

Fig. 4.7 Dissecting aneurysm of the thoracic aorta (arrows). This involves the distal arch and descending aorta (De Bakey Type III). Types I and II involve the ascending aorta and benefit most from surgery. Arrows outline non opacified false lumen.

Angiomatous malformations. These are congenital communications between arteries and veins and are not uncommon. Most of our cases have been in the cerebral circulation (Fig. 4.2), which appears to be one of the common sites for these lesions. They can, however, occur anywhere in the body and arteriography is essential to their localisation and assessment before surgery or embolisation can be undertaken (Fig. 4.8).

Tumours and cysts

Many tumours have a different circulation from the normal tissues around them. In particular malignant tumours are often relatively

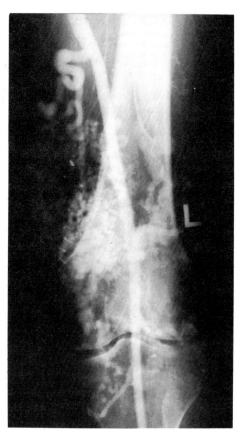

Fig. 4.8   Angiomatous malformation involving the soft tissues above the knee-joints shown by femoral arteriography.

vascular. Arteriography made use of this fact and often enabled tumours in deep-seated organs to be localised. Thus arteriography was for many years vital in the investigation of cerebral tumours. In many cases not only can the tumour be localised by arteriography by showing displacement of normal vessels, but the pattern of the abnormal vessels may prove diagnostic of its pathology.

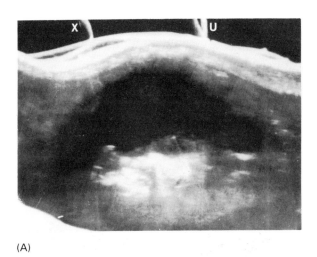

(A)

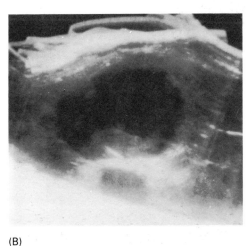

(B)

Fig. 4.9 Aortic aneurysm shown by ultrasound. (A) Longitudinal scan. (B) Transverse scan. X = xiphisternum. U = umbilicus.

With the increasing use of imaging by ultrasound, nuclear medicine, CT and MRI the value of arteriography in the diagnosis of tumours has declined, though it is still used in the assessment of certain tumours for vascularity and malignancy. It is also being increasingly used for tumour treatment by embolisation and for other interventional procedures (see Ch. 13).

Ultrasound

Ultrasound provides a cheap non-invasive and radiation free method of screening elderly patients with suspected abdominal aneurysms (Fig. 4.9). It also enables patients treated conservatively to be easily monitored at regular follow up.

Duplex ultrasound is widely used to screen patients with suspected internal carotid stenosis (Fig. 4.10). Doppler in its various forms is also now used in assessing other vascular stenoses. Colour flow mapping is helpful in assessing abnormal flow patterns within malignant tumours and in differentiating benign lesions such as haemangiomas in organs like the liver.

CT

CT provides another non-invasive method for imaging major vessels and readily demonstrates abdominal aneurysms. It is usual to inject an i.v. bolus of contrast medium prior to the scan to show intraluminal clot or other abnormalities (Fig. 4.11). Dissecting aneurysms can also be diagnosed by CT.

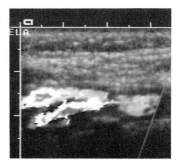

Fig. 4.10 Colour-flow study of a more than 50% stenosis of the common carotid bifurcation and internal carotid origin.

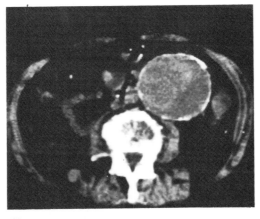

(A)

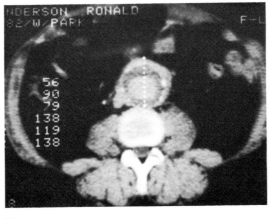

(B)

Fig. 4.11 (A) CT scan of lower abdomen shows a huge abdominal aneurysm with a diameter of 8.5 cm and a calcified wall. (B) CT scan of lower abdomen in another patient after i.v. contrast medium shows the lumen of a medium-sized aneurysm with a wall of clot. The diameter as measured by the electronic cursor is 5.6 cm. The wall is thickened and irregular and enhances with contrast medium, features of so-called 'inflammatory' aneurysms or perianeurysmal fibrosis.

MRI

The absence of intraluminal signal at MRI from rapidly flowing blood provides a high degree of contrast between lumen and vessel wall and surrounding structures, thus making it an excellent method for demonstrating lesions of major vessels (Fig. 4.12).

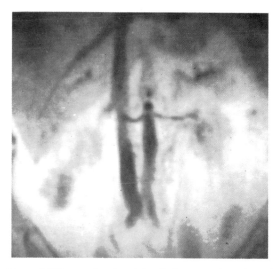

Fig. 4.12   Coronal MR scan showing abdominal aorta and renal arteries, IVC, hepatic and right renal veins.

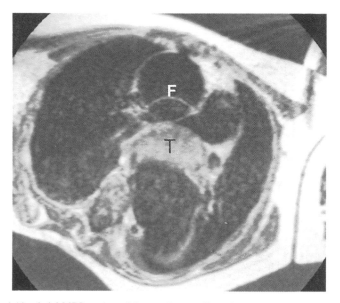

Fig. 4.13   Axial MRI section of thorax shows a dissecting aneurysm. In the ascending aorta both lumens are patent and separated by an intimal flap (F). In the descending aorta the false lumen contains thrombus (T). (Courtesy of Dr Peter Wilde and Bristol MRI Centre.)

Thrombus and haematoma can be differentiated by their relatively high signal (Fig. 4.13). Ultrasound however is so much cheaper and more readily available than MRI that it remains the non-invasive method of choice in most cases. MRI however is increasing in importance in the thorax and brain and for difficult and problem cases not readily resolved by ultrasound, e.g. some cases of dissecting aneurysm and congenital lesions of the major vessels. Recent advances in technique have also greatly improved the resolution and clinical potential of MR angiography (Fig. 4.14).

Veins

Like the arteries these can be demonstrated by most imaging techniques but direct contrast phlebography is still widely used, particularly in the lower limbs for the investigation of suspected deep vein thrombosis. This is particularly important in post-operative patients because of the danger of pulmonary embolus (Fig. 4.15).

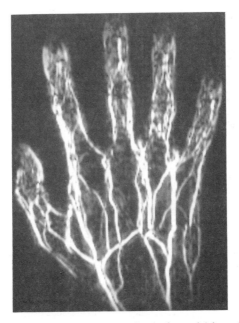

Fig. 4.14 Two dimensional projection gradient refocused (phase shift) MR angiogram of the hand showing vessels as small as 0.2 mm in diameter. (Courtesy of IGE.)

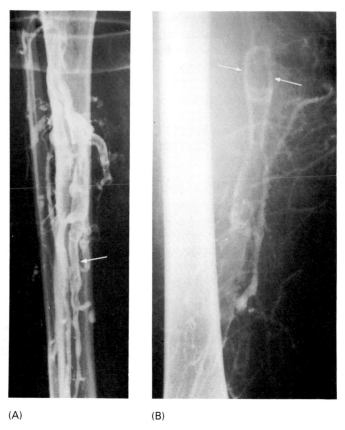

(A)   (B)

Fig. 4.15   Phlebogram showing venous thrombosis in (A) the deep veins of the calf and also in (B) the femoral vein. Clots shown as central filling defects (←).

Many techniques have been elaborated for the assessment of the veins of the lower limb. We use one which requires compression of the superficial veins at the ankle and just below the knee. The contrast injection is made into a vein in the foot and, as the superficial veins are occluded, the contrast is forced into the deep veins. Incompetent communicating veins, however, are outlined as the contrast passes retrogradely through them to the superficial veins.

Inferior vena cavography is performed by percutaneous puncture of one or both femoral veins in the groin. Catheters can also be inserted percutaneously into the femoral veins using the Seldinger technique. Such catheters can be passed upwards into the iliac veins or inferior vena cava. Iliac and inferior vena cavography are used for the investigation of occlusive lesions involving these major veins (Fig. 4.16). Inferior vena cavography has also been widely used in the past for the assessment of para-aortic and retroperitoneal glands involved by reticulosis. Such glands often produce demonstrable defects on the inferior vena cavogram. However, CT is now re-cognised as the most accurate method for assessing abdominal nodes.

Superior vena cavography is performed by passage of the catheter into the median basilic vein at the elbow. In many cases this can be done percutaneously by the use of the Seldinger instrument. Contrast medium is injected at high pressure to demonstrate the innominate veins and superior vena cava. In cases of superior vena

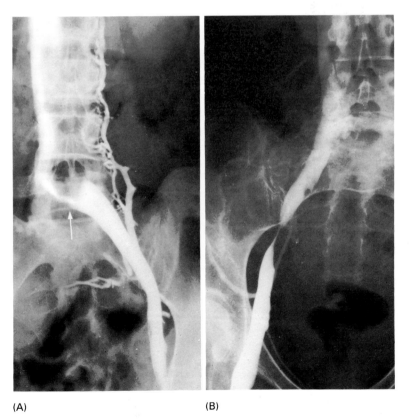

(A)   (B)

Fig. 4.16 (A) Obstruction of the left common iliac vein by pressure from the right common iliac artery (arrow). Note collateral circulation. (B) Iliac vein obstruction by glandular mass.

cava obstruction, the investigation will readily demonstrate the site of the lesion and its extent.

Doppler ultrasound is proving increasingly useful for diagnosing venous thrombosis. Flow signals can be recognised over the femoral, popliteal and calf veins. Deep vein thrombosis is suggested when signals are absent or when muscle compression of the thigh does not produce the expected increase in femoral vein flow. With the addition of *colour flow mapping* a high degree of accuracy is claimed, though smaller lesions in the calf remain difficult to identify.

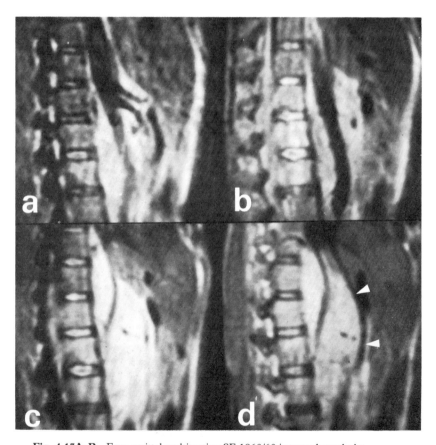

Fig. 4.17A–B   Four sagittal multisection SE 1860/60 images through the abdomen from left (A) to right (D) in a patient with lymphoma. The origins of the coeliac and superior mesenteric arteries are well shown in **A**. In **B** there is anterior displacement of the aorta and in **D** more marked displacement of the inferior vena cava (arrowheads).

CT shows veins well but usually requires contrast injections and is is impractical for routine use. *MRI* also shows major veins well and unlike CT can easily provide coronal and sagittal images (Fig. 4.17). However its high cost and less ready availability remain major disadvantages compared with ultrasound and direct phlebography

C-reactive protein assay is a simple blood test which has a sensitivity of 100% and a specificity of 52% in diagnosing deep

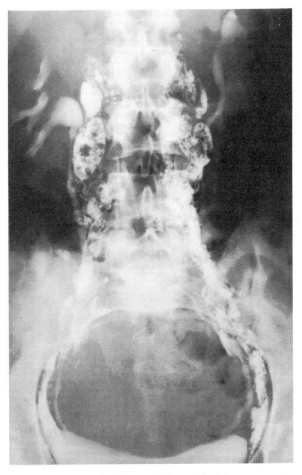

Fig. 4.18 Enlarged para-aortic glands with 'soap bubble' appearance due to Hodgkin's disease. A simultaneous intravenous pyelogram shows early compression of the right ureter just below the renal pelvis.

vein thrombosis. It is therefore a valuable screening test since a normal result excludes deep vein thrombosis and prevents further investigation.

The lymphatic system

Direct lymphangiography was once widely practised but has now been largely superseded by CT in the diagnosis of lymph node lesions and especially neoplasia. Direct lymphangiography involved dissection and cannulation of a lymphatic on the dorsum of the foot followed by slow pump injection of iodised oil. The contrast medium outlines the lymphatics before being taken up by the nodes in the groin, pelvis and abdomen (Fig. 4.18). Normal glands are usually small (less than 1 cm) in diameter whilst glands involved by neoplasia are often markedly enlarged.

CT is non-invasive and is also more accurate than lymphangiography in demonstrating nodal involvement by lymphomas and other neoplasms and is now the investigation of choice in staging tumours (Figs 4.19 and 4.20).

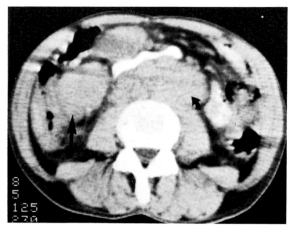

Fig. 4.19 Enlarged para-aortic (curved arrow) and mesenteric (↑) nodes in a case of non-Hodgkin's lymphoma. (The bowel is sandwiched between the enlarged nodes and is opacified by barium (W: 512, L: 35).

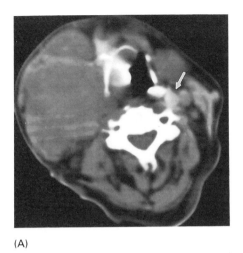

(A)

(B)

Fig. 4.20(A,B) Axial CT sections taken during the injection of i.v. contrast medium. A large malignant nodal mass is seen on the right and extending deep to compress the airway. On the left the dynamic injection of i.v. contrast medium has opacified the vessels of the carotid sheath seen in their normal position (arrow).

5. Bones and joints (Part 1)

Diseases of bones and joints form a large proportion of the work seen in radiological practice. It is clearly impossible to give any but the briefest survey in a work such as this, and that only by omitting important sections. Trauma and fractures are adequately dealt with in standard surgical works and will not therefore be considered. This and the next chapter will be confined to illustrating the value of bone radiology in general medical and surgical problems.

Congenital lesions

There are large numbers of congenital bone lesions and dystrophies and many of these show characteristic radiological appearances. Some are very rare and are of little concern to the student, though they are of considerable interest to the radiologist. A full review of the rarer conditions will be found in monographs or in larger radiology textbooks.

Some bone dystrophies are associated with other lesions and can be diagnosed or suspected on clinical examination as readily as by radiology.

Achondroplasia. The achondroplastic dwarf with large head and trunk and relatively small limbs is easily recognised and was a familiar sight in circuses. *Gargoylism*, or Hurler's syndrome, in its more severe manifestations is also readily diagnosed on clinical inspection. *Osteogenesis imperfecta* can be recognised by the clinician from the characteristic blue sclerotics.

Craniostenosis with premature fusion of the cranial sutures gives rise to characteristic deformity of the skull. The most common variety results in oxycephaly, or turricephaly (Fig. 5.1).

Congenital anomalies of the spine are not rare and may be associated with neurological lesions. In the cervical region, fusion of vertebrae (*Klippel-Feil syndrome*) can occur (Fig. 5.2) and fusion

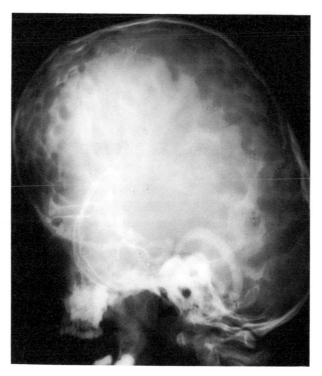

Fig. 5.1   Craniostenosis leading to turricephaly in a child.

of the atlas and occiput (*atlanto-occipital fusion*) is also encountered. In the dorsal region *hemi-vertebrae* are encountered with associated spinal scoliosis and kyphoscoliosis. Severe cases may give rise to kinking of the spinal cord with cord compression. This develops in adolescence as the spine elongates relative to the cord. *Spina bifida* is commonest in the lumbo-sacral region. The gross degrees associated with *syringomyelocele* and *meningomyelocele* are self-evident. In minor degrees the diagnosis can only be made on X-ray, and such minor lesions are often encountered at X-ray as a symptomless chance finding (*spina bifida occulta*).

Congenital anomalies of the limbs are fairly common and include syndactyly, poldactyly and brachydactyly. *Phocomelia* (absence of the proximal parts of the limb) and other severe deformities have been well publicised since the tragic *thalidomide* cases. Attention was focused on these deformities and it was realised that they could be produced by toxic effects *in utero* resulting from drugs taken by the mother. In most of these severe cases radiology does little

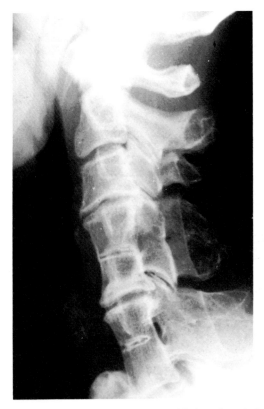

Fig. 5.2   Klippel-Feil syndrome: congenital partial fusion of cervical vertebrae. Rudimentary discs are still present.

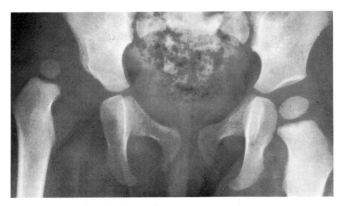

Fig. 5.3   Congenital dislocation of the right hip – note sloping acetabular roof, delayed ossification of the femoral capital epiphysis and false acetabulum formation.

more than emphasise the bony features of an obvious congenital lesion.

Down's syndrome may show characteristic X-ray changes which can be helpful in assessing clinically doubtful cases in infancy. In the hand the middle phalanx of the fifth finger is short and curved and there may be epiphyses at both ends of the metacarpals and metatarsals. The pelvis shows a characteristic appearance with large iliac blades and flat acetabular roofs. There are often only eleven ribs present instead of the normal twelve.

Congenital dislocations. The hip-joint is the only joint at which a congenital dislocation is commonly seen. The diagnosis in infancy was often missed until the child began walking (Fig. 5.3) but careful clinical examination will permit the diagnosis of most cases soon after birth. Once the diagnosis is suspected it can readily be proved or disproved by ultrasound examination. With early diagnosis soon after birth, the results of treatment have been excellent, and the morbidity of this condition much reduced.

Nutritional disorders

Vitamin deficiency. The normal development of bone requires both vitamin C and vitamin D. Deficiency of either of these vitamins in infants will lead on the one hand to scurvy, and on the other to rickets. With improved child welfare both diseases have become rare in this country.

In both cases the radiological appearances are characteristic. In *scurvy* the bone is poorly mineralised and the cortex is thin so that the bone has a 'ground glass' appearance with a fine 'pencilled' cortex. Subperiosteal haemorrhages occur, particularly in the region of the metaphysis, and these are occasionally large (Fig. 5.4).

In infantile *rickets* the bone changes in florid cases are diagnostic. There are considerable growth demands in infant bones and the deficiency of vitamin D results in undermineralisation of newly formed osteoid. Clinically, severe cases show limb deformities and swelling of the weight-bearing epiphyses. Cranio-tabes and the so-called 'rickety rosary' at the costochondral junctions are also seen. On X-ray the broadened epiphysis shows a typical 'saucer' appearance with loss of definition of the metaphysis. The bone as a whole becomes somewhat porotic (Fig. 5.5).

In adults vitamin D deficiency in combination with malnutrition gives rise to *osteomalacia*. This is now rare in Britain but still common in countries where chronic malnutrition is prevalent. It

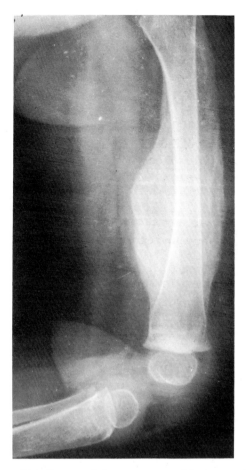

Fig. 5.4 Scurvy. Note the ground glass appearance of the bone and the pencilled outline of the epiphyses. There has been an extensive subperiosteal haemorrhage along the shaft of the femur which has now calcified.

is mainly seen in women and may be associated with, and accentuated by, the calcium drain of pregnancy. The primary defect is again an undermineralisation of osteoid and in severe cases can give rise to gross deformities. The pelvis may become trifoliate and render normal labour impossible, and the discs may herniate into the vertebral bodies ('cod-fish' vertebrae) (Fig. 5.6). Whilst osteomalacia due to dietary deficiency is rarely seen in this country, osteomalacia due to other causes is occasionally encountered. It may be seen in *idiopathic steatorrhoea* or following *coeliac disease*. It may also be encountered in *renal osteodystrophies.*

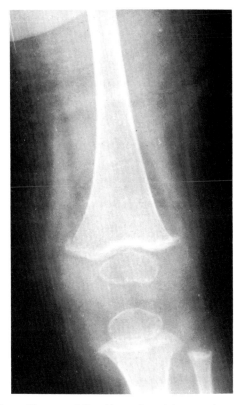

Fig. 5.5   Rickets with saucer deformities at the epiphyses and generalised porosis.

Hypervitaminosis. Overenthusiastic parents will sometimes administer an excess of vitamins to their infants, and cases of hypervitaminosis A and D have been recorded, particularly in the United States. In both cases periostitis may occur and be visible on X-ray. In the case of hypervitaminosis A some osteoporosis may also be seen. With hypervitaminosis D, there may be increased density in the metaphysis.

Metabolic and endocrine disorders

Hyperparathyroidism of the primary type is characterised by true osteoporosis, i.e. there is a quantitative abnormality of the bone in which all the elements including the osteoid are diminished. This is in contrast to osteomalacia in which there is a qualitative defect,

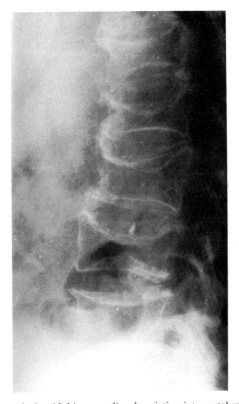

Fig. 5.6 Osteomalacia with biconvex discs herniating into vertebrae.

i.e. osteoid is present but it is not normally mineralised. The osteoporosis of hyperparathyroidism is due to widespread pathological resorption of bone stimulated by overactivity of the parathyroid. An important point is that although the radiological changes can be very severe they are relatively uncommon, occurring in less than 30% of patients. Thus the majority of cases may show no detectable bone changes. When present, however, such changes are fairly characteristic. Apart from the generalised porosis, specific appearances may be seen in the hands where cortical erosions are shown in the phalanges (Fig. 5.7). These are best seen on the radial side of the phalanges and are very characteristic. The skull may also show marked osteoporosis with a diagnostic fine granular appearance ('pepper-pot' skull). There is also some loss of definition between the inner and outer tables and the diploë. An X-ray of the teeth may show loss of the lamina dura or dense cortical line

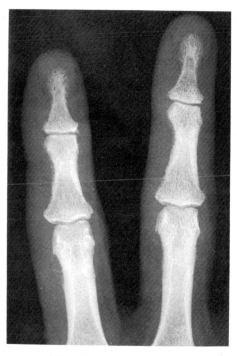

Fig. 5.7   Hyperparathyroidism showing subperiosteal erosion of the lateral aspect of middle phalanges and digital terminal tufts.

of their surrounding bone (Fig. 5.8). Bone cysts due to osteoclastic proliferation may develop late in the disease and deformities of the bone may occur.

In advanced cases deposits of calcium in the kidney substance may occur (*nephrocalcinosis*) and frank renal calculi may develop. All patients with renal calculi and especially patients with recurrent bilateral calculi should be investigated to exclude parathyroid tumours. A single normal serum–calcium level should not be accepted as excluding hyperparathyroidism, and several readings at intervals are now regarded as essential. Estimates of the percentage of patients with renal calculi who are suffering from hyperparathyroidism vary between 5 and 20%.

Secondary hyperparathyroidism may result from chronic renal insufficiency. The consequent disturbance to the normal serum phosphorus and calcium results in parathyroid disturbance. The resulting radiological picture may be very similar to that of primary hyperparathyroidism though cyst formation is unusual.

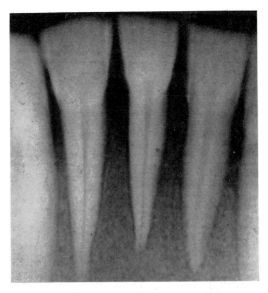

Fig. 5.8 Hyperparathyroidism showing disappearance of the lamina dura, or bony cortex of the tooth sockets.

Hypothyroidism. This gives rise to characteristic changes in infants. *Cretins* have short thick bones. The epiphyses are late in appearing and tend to be irregular and deformed and may be fragmented. There is often a metaphysial band of increased density at the growing ends of the bones (Fig. 5.9).

Cushing's syndrome. Most spontaneous cases are associated with adrenal hyperplasia or tumour. Bone changes consist of osteoporosis affecting mainly the axial skeleton and not the limbs. Painless fractures may occur in the osteoporotic spine and in the ribs and pelvis and these may be discovered by the radiologist though unsuspected clinically. With osteoporosis of the spine there may be collapse and wedging of the vertebral bodies. The characteristic round-shoulder appearance and loss of height in Cushing's syndrome is due to the resulting dorsal kyphosis. With the wide spread use of corticosteroids in the treatment of rheumatic and other disorders, it is important to realise that prolonged *steroid therapy* can induce bone changes identical with those of Cushing's syndrome, even including spinal deformities and spontaneous fractures. Destructive joint changes, particularly in the hips, may also follow steroid therapy (see Ch. 6, p. 103).

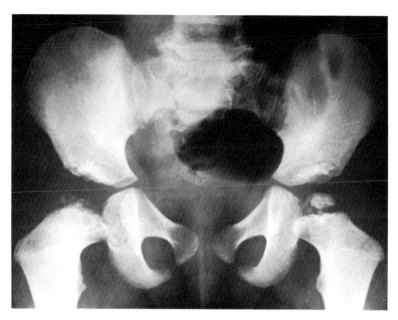

Fig. 5.9   Infantile hypothyroidism showing delayed appearance of femoral head epiphyses with fragmentation in a child of 2½ years. Normally the epiphyses develop in the first year.

Acromegaly. This condition shows characteristic radiological as well as characteristic clinical changes. The skull vault is thickened and the paranasal sinuses are enlarged. The sella is also enlarged in a high proportion of cases. The prognathous mandible is as obvious at X-ray as it is clinically. In bones the muscular attachments are accentuated. The vertebrae become enlarged and kyphosis commonly develops. In the hands the tufts of the terminal phalanges are expanded.

Osteoporosis. The distinction between osteoporosis and osteomalacia has already been emphasised and some of the rare causes such as osteogenesis imperfecta, hyperparathyroidism and Cushing's syndrome have been mentioned. A common form of osteoporosis encountered in clinical practice is so-called *senile osteoporosis.* The exact etiology of this common and often painful disorder remains obscure. Occasionally this type of generalised osteoporosis is seen in younger patients (*pre-senile or idiopathic osteoporosis*). As the osteoporosis progresses, pathological fractures and wedging of the vertebrae are seen, with kyphosis and loss of stature (Fig. 5.10). Since the etiology of senile osteoporosis is not understood, treat-

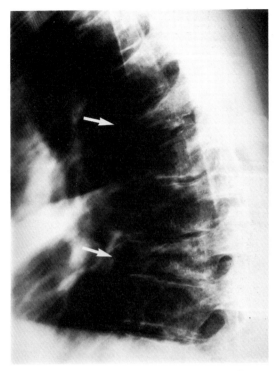

Fig. 5.10 Spinal osteoporosis with spontaneous compression fractures and vertebral wedging (→).

ment is unsatisfactory, and there is as yet no effective therapy for the condition. *Post menopausal osteoporosis* is seen mainly in white females above the age of 50. It is related to reduced oestrogen levels and is commoner in females of slender build.

Paget's disease. The clinical features of the advanced case have been widely recognised since Paget's classic description but the cause of this mysterious and not uncommon disease of bone remains unknown. It is of great interest to the radiologist who often encounters it as a chance finding on routine X-ray of an elderly patient. The pelvis, skull and lumbar spine are perhaps the commonest areas to be involved. The essential bone change is a resorption of the normal bone whilst at the same time new bone is laid down in an abnormal irregular manner. Radiologically, two forms of Paget's disease are recognised and these have been termed the *spongy* and the *amorphous*. The former is the commoner and results in replacement of the normal bone trabeculae by coarse

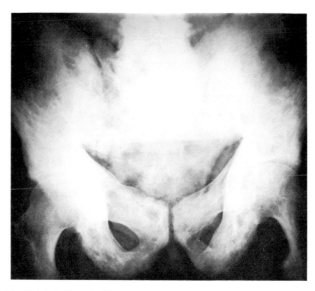

Fig. 5.11   Pelvis in Paget's disease.

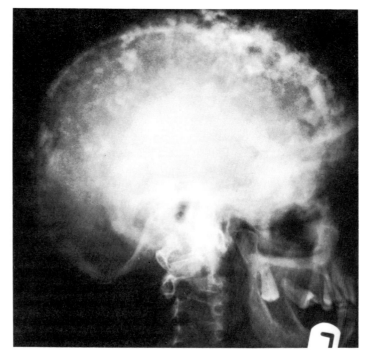

Fig. 5.12   Paget's disease of the skull. The skull vault is thickened with abnormal texture. There is bone softening leading to basilar invagination.

irregular striae (Fig. 5.11). The amorphous type of bone replacement results in a hazy opaque mottled appearance in the bone. Sometimes both processes are seen in the same area. A common feature of Paget's disease is an increase in size and thickness of bone which is very characteristic. When the skull is involved the bone may be three or four times its normal thickness (Fig. 5.12). The skull may also be affected by an unusual type of Paget's disease in which large areas of bone resorption occur (so called *osteoporosis circumscripta*). The femur and tibia are also common sites for Paget's disease but it is rare in the hands or feet. A rare complication of Paget's disease is *sarcoma* developing in an area of affected bone. Most cases of bone sarcoma in elderly patients usually arise in pre-existing Paget's disease.

6. Bones and joints (Part 2)

Inflammatory diseases of bone

With the widespread use of antibiotics, pyogenic infection of bone has become relatively rare except as a result of compound fractures. Further, acute haematogenous osteomyelitis when seen presents a completely different pathological picture from that seen before the advent of antibiotics. Treatment by antibiotics has also profoundly influenced prognosis. Gross destruction of bone with sequestration and chronic sinus formation, which was formerly a major problem, is now rarely seen. In the well-treated case radiological changes may be negligible. In any case it should be remembered that radiological abnormalities in acute osteomyelitis are not detectable for the first week or two of the disease. When antibiotics have been administered from the start and disease is well controlled no bone changes at all may be seen by the radiologist. When treatment has been delayed a periosteal reaction will be demonstrated at the site of the infection together with some osteoporosis of the involved area.

Subacute and chronic osteomyelitis due to invasion with organisms of low-grade virulence may occur in older children and in adults. These can produce destructive bone lesions and give rise to difficulty in differential diagnosis from neoplasm.

Tuberculosis of bone. Tuberculous infection of bones and joints was usually of the bovine type. With the control of bovine tuberculosis now achieved in this country infections of bones and joints are becoming increasingly rare. There has, however, been some recent increase in the incidence and this has been mainly accounted for by immigrants, particularly from the Indian subcontinent. Nevertheless, it is true that cases of tuberculosis of bone and joint which were common in X-ray practice before 1960 are now rarely seen by a general radiologist.

Tuberculous infections of long bones generally produce destructive lesions or can present with so-called 'cystic' manifestations

99

which can cause considerable difficulty in radiological diagnosis. Tuberculosis of the spine (Fig. 6.1) is one of the commonest forms of bone tuberculosis and its onset is usually in infancy or childhood. Characteristically, there is bone destruction and destruction of the intervertebral disc with a resulting fusion of two or more vertebrae and angular kyphosis. Paravertebral cold abscess which may track well away from the bone focus is common. Cord compression may occur from collapse of the vertebrae, or from protrusion of a cold abscess or granulation tissue into the spinal canal.

Syphilis of bone. Like osseous tuberculosis, syphilis of bone is now more commonly seen in radiological museums than in clinical practice. In congenital syphilis radiological evidence of osteochondritis, periostitis, and osteitis is frequent. The metaphysitis is evident in the first months of life, producing a 'saw tooth' or disorganised metaphysis on X-ray. The metaphysis shows increased density with a zone of osteoporosis beneath and metaphysial fracture may occur. These changes are best seen at the knee and wrist.

Skeletal changes may also occur in acquired syphilis, though these are now rarely encountered. In its most characteristic form

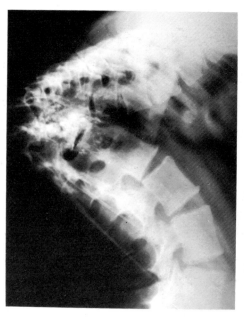

Fig. 6.1 Pott's disease of the spine with fusion of several vertebrae, angular kyphosis and calcified cold abscess.

tertiary syphilis produces a so-called 'lace-work' periostitis, but osteitis with destructive changes is also seen. In the days when it was common tertiary syphilis had the reputation of being the great simulator of other forms of bone disease, so protean were its manifestations.

Arthritis

Acute arthritis due to pyogenic organisms is relatively uncommon. X-ray changes will lag behind the obvious clinical signs in these cases and they are therefore of little help in diagnosis in the early stages. Once cartilage destruction has taken place, infection of bone and sequestration will occur. On recovery there may be irregular sclerosis of the bone around the joint, with fibrous or bony anky-losis. In *acute rheumatic fever* there are no striking X-ray changes although increase in the joint space and soft-tissue swelling may be apparent on X-ray.

Rheumatoid arthritis (Fig. 6.2). In advanced rheumatoid arthritis severe bone and joint changes are demonstrable and these are usually maximal in the hands and feet. The metacarpo-phalangeal

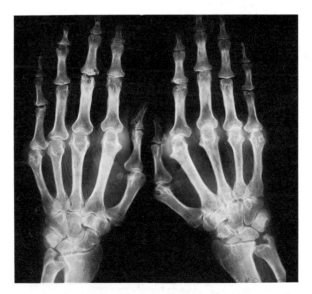

Fig. 6.2   Rheumatoid arthritis showing loss of joint space due to cartilage destruction at metacarpo-phalangeal and interphalangeal joints and small periarticular bone erosions. There is also periarticular osteoporosis.

and proximal interphalangeal joints are mainly affected. There is cartilage destruction with loss of joint space, periarticular bone erosion and subluxation of the joints. Severe loss of cartilage with marked osteoporosis will also be seen in other major joints. In the early cases of rheumatoid arthritis bone changes, though less dramatic, may also be quite diagnostic. In the hands there is usually periarticular porosis of bone, and soft-tissue swelling will be evident around the affected interphalangeal joints. Some loss of cartilage may also be seen.

Tuberculous arthritis (Fig. 6.3). Joint tuberculosis is now rarely seen in Britain except in immigrants. It usually results in destruction of both cartilage and bone around the joint, and in the healing stages goes on to fibrous or bony ankylosis. Radiologically there is periarticular porosis with widening of the joint space in the early stages due to effusion. A destructive focus in the subarticular bone may also be evident. Eventually there is bone destruction on both sides of the joint with little or no evidence of new bone formation.

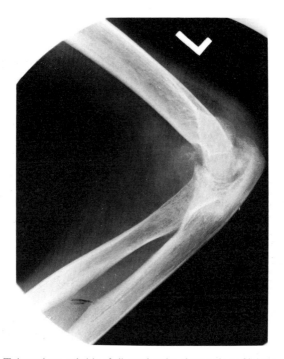

Fig. 6.3 Tuberculous arthritis of elbow showing destruction of joint surface.

An old healed tuberculous joint may be ankylosed and show alteration in the trabecular pattern around the joint.

Steroid therapy can give rise to a destructive arthritis in the hip (Fig. 6.4). This may be due to the pain of minor trauma being masked by the steroids and leading to avascular necrosis.

Gout

In this predominantly male disease the X-ray changes are not seen until the disease has been present for some time. The most characteristic changes are seen in the hands and feet. Classically, small areas of bone are eroded at the articular margins due to deposits of sodium biurate and these have a 'punched out' appearance on X-ray (Fig. 6.5). Deposits may also appear in the soft tissues and these may calcify.

Osteoarthrosis

Large joints are mainly affected, particularly the hips and knees,

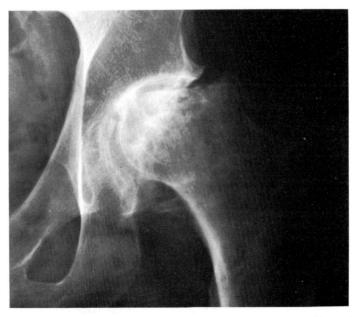

Fig. 6.4 Destructive arthritis of the hip following avascular necrosis of femoral head due to steroid therapy.

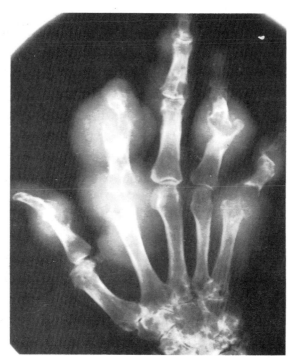

Fig. 6.5 Advanced gout, showing punched out periarticular erosions with soft tissue swellings.

though the condition also occurs in other joints. Age and trauma seem to be the main predisposing factors. Heredity may also be important.

Radiologically the appearances are characteristic. First, there is loss of cartilage appearing as a narrowing of the joint space. Then subarticular bone sclerosis occurs, sometimes with 'pseudo cyst' formation adjacent to the joint. 'Lipping' or bony extensions around the margins of the joint are also seen. When there is gross loss of cartilage, pain and disability may be severe, particularly in the hip (Fig. 6.6). Orthopaedic surgery may eventually be necessary and hip replacements are now commonplace.

Disc degeneration

Spinal disc degeneration is common with increasing age. The clinical manifestations are well known and the so-called 'slipped

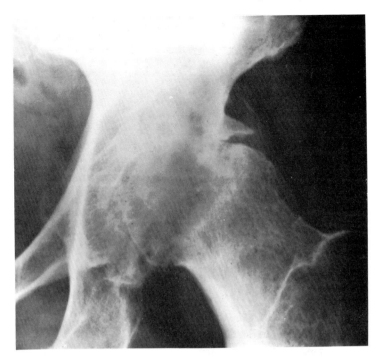

Fig. 6.6 Severe osteoarthrosis of the hip.

disc' is now well recognised by the lay public as the common cause of sciatica. The acute lesion in the younger patient may show little on X-ray of the spine except narrowing of the affected disc space. In the more long-standing cases there is usually sclerosis of the bone and osteoarthritic lipping around the narrowed disc space.

In the cervical region disc degeneration shows similar changes of narrowing of the disc space, adjacent bony sclerosis and osteo-arthritic lipping (Fig. 6.7). The clinical manifestations are *brachial neuritis* with pain and limitation of movement in the neck and shoulder muscles, or long tract signs. Whilst cervical disc degener-ation is the common cause of this syndrome it is important to realise that severe disc degeneration may be shown on X-ray in patients with little in the way of clinical symptoms. The radiological findings must therefore always be interpreted in the light of the clinical picture.

Most disc lesions are diagnosed on the clinical history and plain X-rays. However, when surgery is being considered more complex

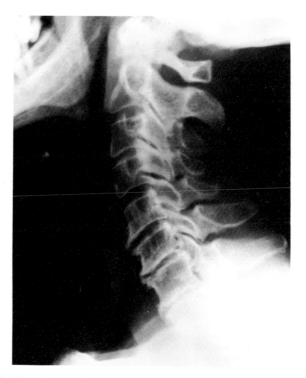

Fig. 6.7 Disc degeneration and osteoarthritis of the cervical spine. Note narrowing of disc spaces and adjacent bony lipping from C5 to D1.

investigation is usually required by myelography, computed myelography (CM), or MRI.

Perthes' disease, or osteochondritis of the femoral head, starts in children between the age of five and ten and is more common in boys than girls. There is local pain with limitation of movement in the affected hip. In the classical case radiology shows the diagnostic appearance of flattening, fragmentation and condensation of the femoral head and epiphysis (Fig. 6.8). After healing the femoral neck is thickened and the head deformed.

Neuropathic joints show a characteristic appearance on X-ray. In the lower limb such 'Charcot' joints are usually due to *tabes dorsalis* and are most commonly seen at the hip or knee. The joint may become completely disorganised with destruction of the joint surface, sclerosis of the underlying bone and calcareous debris around. In the hip it is not uncommon for the whole femoral head and neck to disappear. The lumbar spine may also be involved in tabes and there is often marked narrowing of the joint spaces with

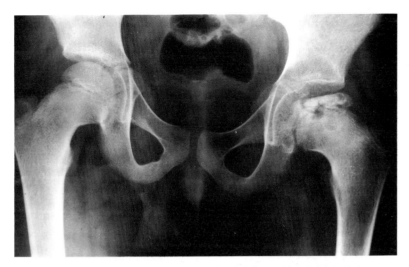

Fig. 6.8 Perthes' disease of the hip joint. The left femoral head epiphysis is flattened, fragmented and condensed.

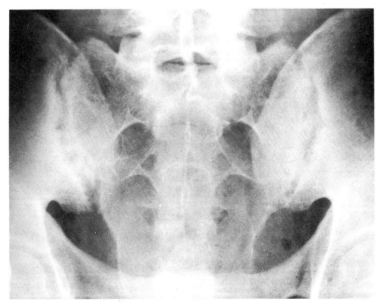

(A)

Fig. 6.9(A) Caption see overleaf.

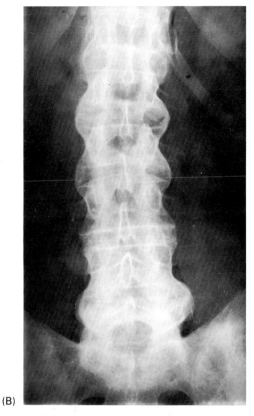

(B)

Fig. 6.9 Ankylosing spondylitis. (A) Fusion of SI joints. (B) Lumbar spine showing bamboo appearance due to ossification of ligaments.

exuberant bony osteophytosis and bony sclerosis. Charcot joints in the upper limb are usually due to *syringomyelia* and here again there may be gross disorganisation of the joint with little or no pain. The X-ray appearances are usually diagnostic.

Ankylosing spondylitis is a disease mainly affecting young men, although older men and even women are not immune. Advanced cases show the characteristic 'bamboo spine' due to ossification of the longitudinal spinal ligaments (Fig. 6.9B). Earlier changes are 'squaring' of the vertebral bodies with loss of their normal anterior concavity. The earliest X-ray changes in this condition, however, are to be found in the sacro-iliac joints. The margins of the joints become irregular and serrated and the joints become narrowed with sclerosis of the subjacent iliac bone (Fig. 6.9A).

Primary tumours of bone

Primary benign tumours of bone are often encountered as chance findings on routine radiology. They include simple bone cysts (usually seen in children and young adults), enchondromas, simple osteomas, and osteochondromas. Simple bone cysts sometimes present with pathological fracture.

Primary malignant tumours of bone include osteogenic sarcoma, chondrosarcoma, Ewing's tumour, malignant osteoclastoma and other rarer tumours.

Osteogenic sarcoma, in which the prognosis is so grave, occurs mainly in children or adolescents, although it is also encountered in elderly patients as a complication of Paget's disease. The radiological manifestations can differ widely. Some tumours are markedly osteolytic (Fig. 6.10A) producing widespread bone destruction; others are markedly osteoblastic, producing irregular bone sclerosis (Fig. 6.10B). X-ray appearances are often diagnostic with 'sun-ray' spicules of bone extending out into the soft tissues and a characteristic periosteal reaction at the margin of the tumour (Codman's triangle). In both cases there may be involvement of soft tissues with extension of the tumour outside the bone. CT or MRI shows

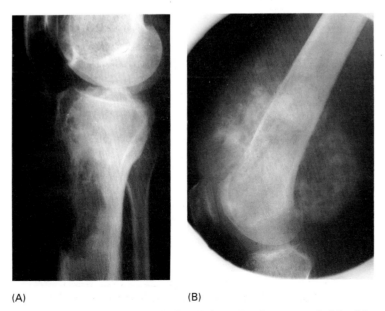

(A)   (B)

Fig. 6.10   Osteogenic sarcoma. (A) Osteolytic type, at the upper end of the tibia. (B) Sclerosing type with calcification extending into the soft tissues.

this well. Metastases usually occur in the lung and can be of the large 'cannon ball' variety.

Multiple myeloma occurs mainly in middle-aged and elderly patients and the diagnosis is often missed in the early stages. Clinically, bone pain and generalised weakness may be presenting features. The X-ray appearances are often diagnostic although marrow puncture and electrophoresis may be necessary to confirm the diagnosis. Myelomatous deposits appear as small punched-out holes in the bone. Characteristically these involve the inner surface of the cortex in the long bones. Sometimes, particularly in the spine, an appearance is produced resembling generalised osteo-porosis. Small round punched-out deposits are also seen in the skull and are virtually diagnostic (Fig. 6.11).

Osteoid osteoma. Despite its name, osteoid osteoma is not really a tumour. This interesting condition often gives rise to severe local bone pain. Radiology shows a small localised bony sclerosis with a central translucent area or 'nidus'. It is characteristic of these patients that for some unexplained reason the severe pain is often relieved by aspirin.

Metastatic tumours

The bony skeleton is a common site for metastases, and secondary

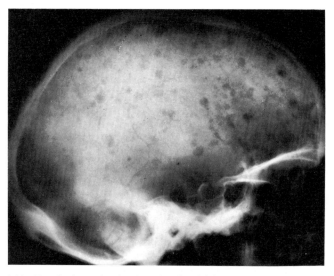

Fig. 6.11 Punched-out circular deposits of multiple myeloma in the skull vault.

deposits are commonly seen in carcinoma of the breast, carcinoma of the lung and other forms of malignancy. Metastases in bone may show quite varied radiological appearances. They may produce purely *osteolytic* lesions or they may produce an *osteoblastic* reaction. Mixed osteolytic and osteoblastic deposits are also seen, since it is possible for the same primary carcinoma to produce both osteolytic and osteoblastic secondary deposits. In most types of tumour, however, the deposits tend to be predominantly of one type. Thus, carcinoma of the kidney nearly always produces osteolytic deposits, whereas carcinoma of the prostate or pancreas commonly produces osteoblastic deposits. The widespread involvement of bone by metastases, which occurs in the terminal stages of many carcinomas, is

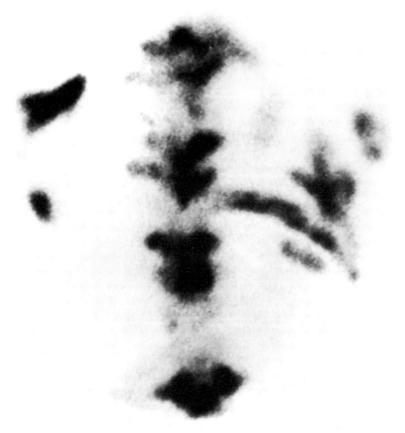

Fig. 6.12 Bone metastases showing as areas of high uptake in the vertebrae, ribs and scapulae.

associated with pain, weakness and severe anaemia. Bone involved by metastases may undergo pathological fracture, and patients may occasionally present with a spontaneous fracture. X-rays will show that this is a pathological fracture and a previously unsuspected malignancy will be diagnosed.

Isotope scanning

Bone scanning in the form of *total body imaging* is now widely practised in the assessment of metastatic spread from carcinoma. Phosphate complexes labelled with $^{99}Tc^m$ are generally used and

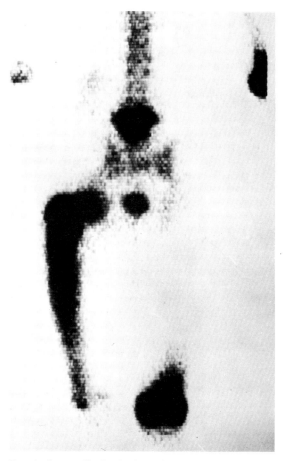

Fig. 6.13 Paget's disease affecting both the femora and other bones.

are taken up by many bone lesions (Figs 6.12 and 6.13). It is more accurate in picking up bone secondaries than the simple radiological skeletal survey and is widely used for this purpose. However, it should be realised that positive bone scans are non-specific and are found with most benign lesions of bone as well as with malignant lesions. These include Paget's disease, fibrous dysplasia, bone fractures, and inflammatory bone lesions, as well as osteoarthritis and rheumatoid arthritis. It is vital therefore that bone scans should always be interpreted in relation to X-ray studies taken at about the same time.

The most widely used bone scanning agent is now $^{99}Tc^m$ diphosphate.

7. Gastroenterology (Part 1)

Salivary glands

Radiology may be required in the investigation of salivary gland swellings.

Calculi are commoner in the submandibular than in the parotid gland. They are usually found in the duct but can occur in the gland itself. The latter tend to be rounded whilst those in the duct are

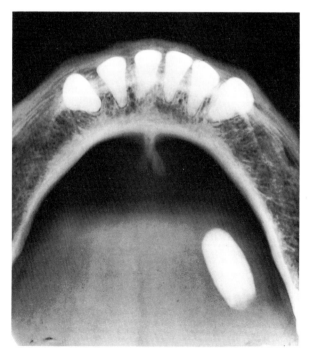

Fig. 7.1   Intra-oral view of the submandibular duct showing a large oval salivary calculus lodged in the duct.

elongated. They vary in length from a few millimetres to a centimetre or more, and can usually be identified on simple radiographs, as some 80% are radiopaque (Fig. 7.1).

Submandibular calculi may have to be differentiated from calcified cervical glands or from islands of bone sclerosis in the mandible when the latter is superimposed on the duct.

Sialography is performed by injecting either the parotid or submaxillary duct using a fine cannula; 1–2 ml of a viscous or water soluble contrast medium are used. The procedure will demonstrate a non opaque calculus. It will also show strictures of the ducts and post-obstructive or post-inflammatory sialectasis.

Sialography shows merely displacement of ducts and intraglandular branches in the benign tumours (Fig. 7.2) but gross distortion and invasion of the ducts may be seen in carcinoma.

Tumours of the salivary glands are usually *mixed salivary tumours*, but *carcinomas* are sometimes seen and mixed salivary tumours may become malignant after inadequate surgical removal. They are best assessed by CT (Fig. 7.3) or by MRI.

Pharynx and oesophagus

Examination of the pharynx and oesophagus by the radiologist is usually performed as a routine at all barium meal examinations,

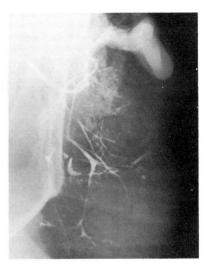

Fig. 7.2 Mixed salivary tumour showing distortion of gland ducts at sialogram (tangential view).

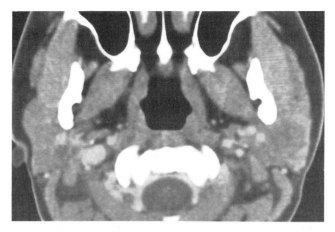

Fig. 7.3 Parotid adenocarcinoma, post-contrast examination: irregularly enhancing mass in the left parotid showing obliteration of the subcutaneous fat and deep extension medial to the ramus of the mandible. Compare normal gland on right.

even when examination of the stomach and not the oesophagus is requested. In this way unsuspected cases of diaphragmatic hernia and gastro-oesophageal regurgitation are detected, and occasionally more important lesions such as achalasia and even carcinoma are encountered.

Dysphagia. The commonest indication for requesting an X-ray examination of the oesophagus alone is dysphagia. Among the organic causes demonstrated by radiology are:

1. Swallowed foreign body
2. Pharyngeal pouch
3. Pharyngeal neuromuscular incoordination associated with bulbar and pseudobulbar palsy
4. Achalasia of the cardia, and other forms of neuromuscular incoordination
5. Carcinoma
6. Plummer–Vinson syndrome
7. Hiatus hernia and/or reflux oesophagitis.

Functional dysphagia may be encountered, particularly in young women, and radiology plays an important part in excluding an organic cause. Careful radiological examination is essential since many cases considered to be 'functional' are later proved to have organic disease.

Pharyngeal pouch. This condition is seen most frequently in elderly male patients and may present with dysphagia or food regurgitation. The appearances are quite characteristic. The pouch projects backwards and downwards from the posterior aspect of the pharyngo-oesophageal junction. At this point there is a gap (Killian's dehiscence) between the transverse and oblique fibres of the inferior constriction of the pharynx (Fig. 7.4).

Foreign body. Whilst an impacted foreign body may be readily identified radiologically, fish bones, and even small chicken and rabbit bones can sometimes be most difficult to identify. Using a careful technique, however, most impacted foreign bodies can be demonstrated by the radiologist.

Neuromuscular incoordination received much radiological attention when the image intensifier and cine-radiology made possible careful analysis of cine-films of the mechanism of swallowing. Similar studies have thrown much light on the complex mechanism of normal swallowing.

Achalasia of the cardia has a characteristic appearance on

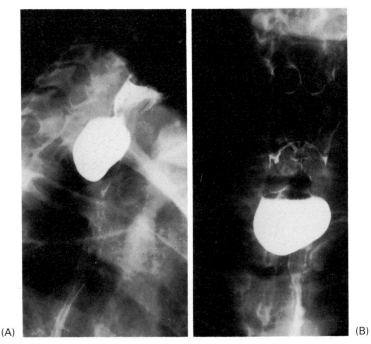

(A)　　　　　　　　　　　　　　　　　　　　　　　(B)

Fig. 7.4 Pharyngeal pouch lateral and AP views showing forward displacement of the oesophagus by the distended diverticulum.

screening (see Fig. 7.5). The oesophagus is grossly dilated and may contain fluid and food debris, or even a fluid level, in a fasting patient. The dilated oesophagus may be seen on a plain X-ray of the chest lateral to the right heart border, and rendered opaque by the contained fluid and food debris. In the classical case the obstruction at the cardia tapers smoothly in the so-called 'rat's tail' manner. Another fairly constant feature is absence of the normal gas bubble in the cardia of the stomach. In addition to spasm at the cardia cine studies or video fluoroscopy show gross disorder of the whole neuro-muscular mechanism of swallowing and therefore of the normal propulsion of food down the dilated oesophagus.

Carcinoma of the oesophagus usually occurs at one of three sites:

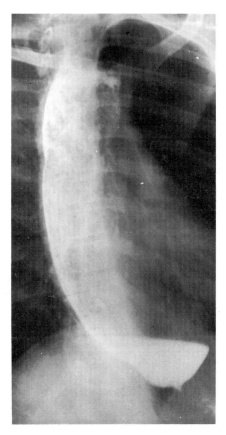

Fig. 7.5   Achalasia showing grossly dilated oesophagus with pool of barium at its lower end.

the lower end, the upper end, or the middle third opposite the aortic arch. In most cases radiological diagnosis presents little difficulty (see Fig. 7.6). Occasionally differential diagnosis between a neoplasm at the lower end of the oesophagus and achalasia can present a problem, particularly in elderly patients. The same is true of strictures with peptic oesophagitis and hiatus hernia.

Oesophageal webs due to mucosal folds may be demonstrated in association with the dysphagia encountered in the *Plummer–Vinson syndrome*. These lesions are important because they were once thought to be pre-cancerous, though this is now less certain. Thus patients with sideropenic anaemia and dysphagia must be kept under careful observation. Oesophageal webs are best demons-

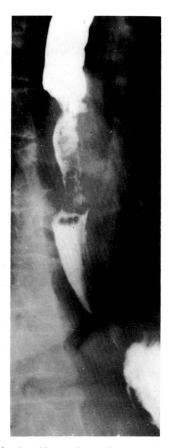

Fig. 7.6 Irregular defect in mid-oesophagus due to carcinoma.

trated by cine-films or video fluoroscopy of barium swallows obtained with the aid of an image intensifier. The web appears as a thin horizontal linear band defect extending back from the anterior wall and sometimes causes partial obstruction.

Oesphageal varices, as a complication of cirrhosis of the liver and portal hypertension, may give rise to severe haematemesis, and examination of the oesophagus for varices is often requested in patients with cirrhosis, or with unexplained haematemesis. In some cases diagnosis is obvious and the wormlike impressions on the barium of large submucosal varices are readily identified (Fig. 7.7). In other cases a most meticulous radiological examination, including mucosal films of the oesophagus taken with the patient performing the Valsalva manoeuvre, or other manoeuvres to dilate the veins,

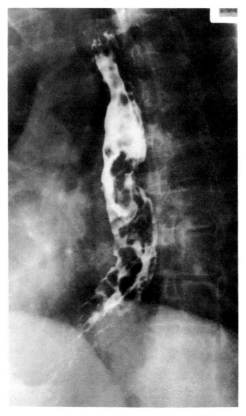

Fig. 7.7   Oesophageal varices producing worm-like impressions.

may fail to show them. A negative barium swallow examination therefore does not exclude oesophageal varices.

Hiatus hernia. Lesions of the lower end of the oesophagus, and in particular hiatus hernia, are common (Fig. 7.8). Diagnosis of the major degree of hiatus hernia with a large intra-thoracic loculus is straightforward, but the diagnosis of a small degree of sliding hernia may require a careful radiological technique with studies in the Trendelenberg position. A plain chest film may show a large hiatus hernia as a ring shadow containing a fluid level and superimposed on the cardiac shadow (Fig. 7.9).

Gastro-oesophageal regurgitation will also require careful examination by the radiologist for its demonstration.

Peptic oesophagitis. Both hiatus hernia and gastro-oesophageal regurgitation may be associated with peptic oesophagitis (Fig. 7.8). In its more advanced form peptic oesophagitis will lead to an elongated stricture of the oesophagus. A small ulcer crater may, or may not, be demonstrated.

Stomach and duodenum

Peptic ulcer. Chronic peptic ulcers are among the commoner lesions demonstrated during examination of the stomach and

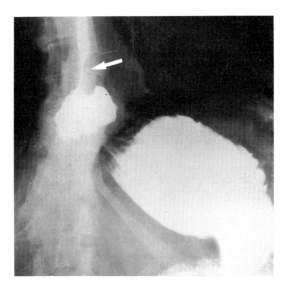

Fig. 7.8 Small hiatus hernia with oesophageal reflux and peptic oesophagitis. Note the narrowed lower end of the oesophagus (←).

duodenum. Usually the clinical evidence and the radiological appearances are characteristic but sometimes problems of differential diagnosis arise. One of the most important problems for the radiologist is the differentiation between a large chronic benign ulcer of the stomach (Fig. 7.10) and a *malignant ulcer* in the middle-aged or elderly patient.

Whilst there are various radiological signs which assist the radiologist to come to a decision, e.g. the relationship of the ulcer to the gastric lumen, the presence or absence of a beaded edge, motility of the adjacent stomach area, response to simple therapy – it is important to realise that it may be quite impossible for a radiologist to be dogmatic as to whether an ulcer is benign or malignant. In these cases laparotomy was once the only means of deciding, though, today in skilled hands, endoscopy and biopsy will usually settle the issue. Chronic duodenal ulcers are less of a problem in this respect as malignancy in the duodenum is rare. Occasionally, however, *pyloric obstruction* produced by the chronic cicatrisation associated with a duodenal ulcer may have to be differentiated from the pyloric obstruction of malignancy.

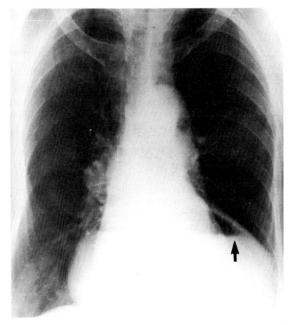

Fig. 7.9   Hiatus hernia shown as huge circular mass with fluid level (↑) superimposed on the heart shadow.

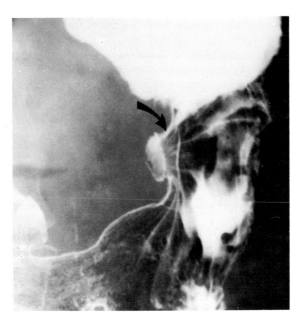

Fig. 7.10 Large benign gastric ulcer demonstrated in profile. The ulcer crater projects outside the wall of the stomach and mucosal folds extend to the edge of the crater.

Benign ulcers are relatively rare on the greater curvature and lesions here or in the prepyloric region should be regarded with suspicion. Multiple peptic ulcers are occasionally seen, and the possibility of the Zollinger–Ellison syndrome should then be considered. This is due to a 'β' *cell tumour* of the pancreas. Such patients may also show a malabsorption pattern in the small bowel (see below).

In the past there has been a tendency to abuse the assessment of healing of gastric ulcers by radiological methods. It is certainly not necessary for a patient who is clinically well to continue to have regular periodic examinations of his stomach and duodenum to make sure that an ulcer remains healed completely. On the other hand, radiological control is always helpful when clinical doubt as to healing persists.

Carcinoma of the stomach may present in other forms besides that of malignant ulcer. Diffuse infiltration of the gastric wall may occur giving rise to rigidity and localised contraction (Fig. 7.11). Infiltration of the whole gastric wall can give rise to the malignant form of *linitis plastica*. Large polypoid or encephaloid carcinomas may also occur in the stomach (Fig. 7.12). If these are in the region

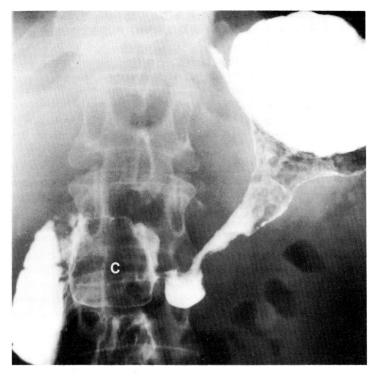

Fig. 7.11   Scirrhous carcinoma of stomach showing narrowed lumen. Almost all of the stomach is involved. C = duodenal cap.

of the fundus they can sometimes be missed unless the area is very carefully examined. Carcinoma of the fundus of the stomach may also involve the cardia and present with lower oesophageal obstruction. Prepyloric carcinomas may present with pyloric stenosis. Thus, whilst carcinoma of the stomach can be one of the easiest lesions for a radiologist to diagnose, it can also be one of the most difficult and require careful double contrast mucosal studies.

CT is valuable in the staging of gastric carcinoma. It can show direct spread to the liver, pancreas and mesentery as well as nodal and liver metastases and spread to the peritoneal cavity.

Benign tumours of the stomach are not uncommon in radiological practice. *Leiomyoma* is probably the most frequently encountered, and other benign tumours are sometimes seen including neurilemmoma, fibroma and lipoma. These benign tumours usually present as a large rounded defect in the stomach. They may contain a small central crater, where the mucosa has ulcerated. Their appearance

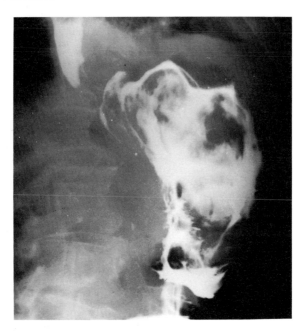

Fig. 7.12 Encephaloid carcinoma in fundus and body of stomach producing large irregular filling defects.

is fairly typical and can usually be differentiated from that of an encephaloid carcinoma.

Duodenal ulcer. Duodenal ulcer is among the most common lesions seen by radiologists (Fig. 7.13). The normal duodenal cap fills out well with barium and appears as a regular cone or inverted acorn. Ulcers are usually demonstrated on the anterior or posterior surface as 'niches' which the radiologist attempts to show both 'en face' and in profile. Sometimes there is considerable oedema around the ulcer and this may produce a small rounded filling defect in the cap. In cases in which an ulcer crater is difficult to fill, either from oedema or because it is shallow, there are ancillary radiological signs to suggest duodenal ulceration. These include spasm and constant deformity of the cap, fleeting filling of the cap, pyloric spasm, evidence of increased peristaltic activity in the stomach, and tenderness on palpation of the cap. Like the radiological control of the healing of gastric ulcer, radiological observation of healing of duodenal ulcers has tended to be abused in the past. Once a duodenal ulcer is diagnosed the necessity for repeated examinations should be critically examined in the light of the clinical progress.

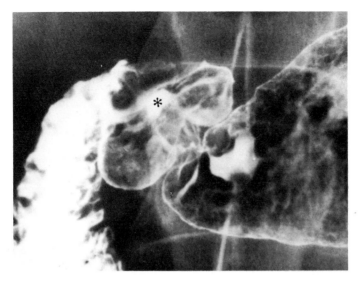

Fig. 7.13   Duodenal cap with a central ulcer crater (*).

Tumours of the duodenum are much rarer than tumours of the stomach. Examination of the duodenum is however important in the assessment of suspected cases of carcinoma of the head of the pancreas and of carcinoma of the ampulla of Vater. In carcinoma of the head of the pancreas the duodenal loop may be widened and expanded, and the medial border of the second part of the duodenum may show Frostberg's 'inverted 3' sign.

Hypotonic duodenography. In this technique the patient is given a small dose of glucagon (0.1 mg) during his barium meal. This temporarily inhibits all peristalsis in the duodenum and allows double contrast films of the dilated duodenal loop to be obtained showing its outlines very clearly. In this way small irregularities, e.g. those due to involvement by a carcinoma of the head of the pancreas, are better shown.

Duodenal ileus is sometimes encountered as a result of pressure of the mesentery on the third part of the duodenum giving rise to partial obstruction. It occurs particularly in debilitated patients being nursed in the supine position. Duodenal ileus may also accompany acute or subacute pancreatitis.

Duodenal diverticula. Small diverticula are often detected as a chance finding in the second and third parts of the duodenum. They may also be found in the proximal jejunum. Symptoms, however, are unusual unless the diverticula are widespread.

Small bowel

The radiological technique for examination of the small bowel has in the past consisted of the 'follow-through meal'. Barium given by mouth is observed passing through the small bowel by repeated screening and films taken over a period of several hours. This is clearly a tedious and time-consuming method of investigation and, so far as small lesions are concerned, it is somewhat 'hit and miss'.

Attempts were therefore made to improve the situation by the development of special techniques of *small bowel enema.*

With experience, tubes can be readily passed into the duodenum with little discomfort to the patient, and by the use of appropriate contrast media, films can be obtained of the whole of the small bowel within a period of twenty to thirty minutes. Simpler methods of obtaining rapid filling of the small bowel include getting the patient to lie on his right side and drink iced water, or administering drugs such as metoclopramide.

Tumours of the small bowel are relatively uncommon, and most cases present with small bowel obstruction.

Small intestinal malabsorption. A common clinical indication for examination of the small bowel is suspicion of small intestinal malabsorption. A fairly characteristic picture has been described in a number of conditions: e.g. idiopathic steatorrhoea, sprue, coeliac disease, mesenteric disease. This consisted mainly of *dilatation* of the small bowel, and sometimes of *clumping* of the barium in irregular puddles in contrast to the normal regular pattern (Fig. 7.14 A and B). The appearances can be simulated by non-pathological conditions in certain circumstances but the radiologist can usually differentiate between the pathological and the variants of normal by using non-flocculating solutions of barium, such as Raybar.

The radiologist classifies malabsorption syndromes into two different groups:

1. Lesions mainly those of steatorrhoea
2. Lesions with specific features.

The causes may be listed as in Table 7.1.

Crohn's disease, or regional enteritis, in its classical form affects the terminal ileum (Fig. 7.15) and gives rise to the characteristic radiological picture of a stenosed channel replacing the distal segment of the ileum (the so-called 'string sign'). The disease, however, is not confined to the ileum and may affect any portion of the bowel. Clinically the condition is often mistaken for acute or chronic appendicitis.

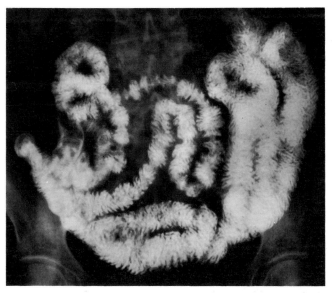

(A)

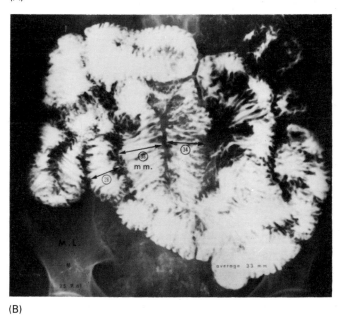

(B)

Fig. 7.14   A. Normal small bowel showing continuous feathery pattern of the small intestine. **B.** Adult coeliac disease. Moderate dilatation of jejunum in a patient with diarrhoea due to steatorrhoea. Biopsy showed subtotal villous atrophy. Normal small bowel is less than 25 mm in diameter.

Table 7.1 Malabsorption (after Laws)

Group 1 — Features mainly of steatorrhoea
  A. *Diffuse lesions of mucosa*
    Coeliac disease
    Idiopathic steatorrhoea (adult coeliac disease, or gluten-induced enteropathy)
    Tropical sprue
    Infiltrations: Whipple's disease
              amyloidosis
  B. *Defects of digestion*
    (a) Deficiency of bile
        Obstructive jaundice
        Biliary cirrhosis
    (b) Deficiency of pancreatic enzymes
        Cystic fibrosis
        Chronic pancreatitis
        Pancreatectomy
  C. Post-gastrectomy steatorrhoea

Group 2 — Conditions with specific radiological features
  A. *Localised (often multiple) lesions of the small intestine*
    Regional ileitis
    Hodgkin's disease
    Lymphosarcoma
    Diffuse sclerosis (scleroderma)
  B. *Anatomical lesions of the small intestine*
    (a) Resection
        Proximal resection
        Distal resection
    (b) Bacterial contamination
        Jejunal diverticulosis
        Stagnant loop
        Ileal stricture
        Fistula
    (c) Mixed lesions (resection plus bacterial contamination)
  C. *Disaccharidase deficiency*
    Hypolactasia
    Hyposucrasia

Chronic appendicitis. The radiological diagnosis of chronic appendicitis was often made at one time but most observers now regard a radiological diagnosis of chronic appendicitis with scepticism. The alleged radiological signs of chronic appendicitis were non-filling or incomplete filling of the appendix at a follow-through barium meal, the presence of calculi in the appendix, fixation and tenderness of the appendix and barium stasis in the appendix. It has been shown that these signs are found as often among those with healthy appendices as among those with diseased organs. If a diagnosis of chronic appendicitis is to be made it should be made on clinical not radiological grounds. Radiology, however, is useful in demonstrating other pathological lesions in this region simulating chronic appendicitis. It will, for instance, provide a positive

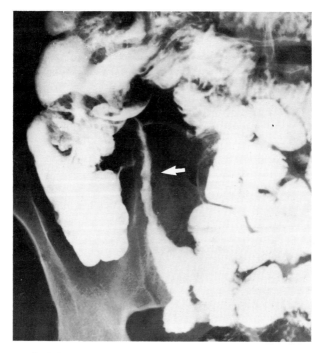

Fig. 7.15 Crohn's disease showing marked narrowing of the terminal ileum (←).

diagnosis in such conditions as regional enteritis, ileo-caecal tuberculosis, and appendix abscess.

Disaccharidase deficiency. Vague abdominal symptoms and diarrhoea may occur in this condition which is usually due to lactase deficiency and more rarely to sucrase deficiency. The diagnosis can be confirmed by adding 25 g of the test sugar to the barium meal. The diagnostic features are then marked dilution of the barium in the small bowel so that the whole of the bowel is filled with the dilute mixture and the coils appear rather dilated. The mixture reaches the colon very rapidly and the colon also fills rapidly with dilute barium.

8. Gastroenterology (Part 2)

Large bowel

If disease of the large bowel is suspected then it is essential that a barium enema be performed since examination of the large bowel by follow-through technique following an oral barium meal will fail to demonstrate a high proportion of colonic lesions. Such an examination should never be accepted as excluding abnormality of the large bowel when the symptoms suggest that a colonic lesion is present.

Before a barium enema is performed it is essential that the whole colon should be cleared of faecal material and thoroughly

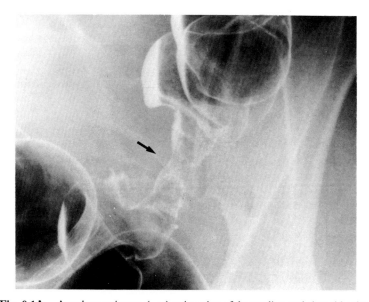

Fig. 8.1A. Annular carcinoma (→) at junction of descending and sigmoid colon.

133

cleansed by adequate colonic lavage, preferably using the Studa chair method and normal saline for irrigation. The single-contrast barium enema was routinely used for many years, but has now been largely replaced by the technique of barium enema popularised by Swedish workers. The so-called Malmö technique has greatly increased the diagnostic accuracy of the barium enema and enables even small polyps in the colon to be detected at an early stage. It necessitates not only thorough cleansing of the large bowel but also routine *double-contrast* visualisation of the colon throughout its course. This is achieved by air distension of the barium-coated mucosa.

The common clinical indications for barium enema are *diarrhoea, alterations in the bowel habit,* the presence of an *abdominal mass* suspected as colonic, *melaena,* or suspected *colonic obstruction.*

Carcinoma of the large bowel is usually annular in type and on barium enema appears as a localised stenosing lesion, showing a characteristic 'napkin ring' deformity (Fig. 8.1A). Encephaloid

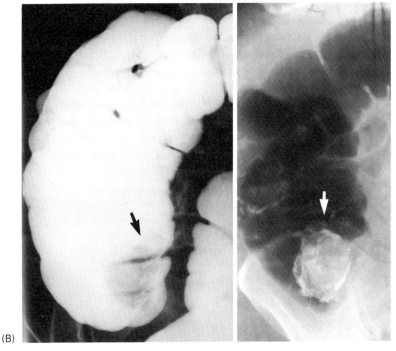

(B)

(C)

Fig. 8.1B & C   Carcinoma of the caecum shown (B) by single-contrast barium enema and largely masked by barium; (C) clearly demonstrated by double-contrast enema.

carcinomas are less common. In the caecum, however, they can present as large irregular filling defects (Fig. 8.1B and C). It is important to realise that the barium enema can easily miss a carcinoma in the rectum where the lesion is obscured in the dilated and barium-filled cavity. Carcinoma of the rectum should be diagnosed by digital examination or proctoscopy. Nevertheless most experienced radiologists have encountered cases at barium enema, which the referring physician has missed because of inadequate examination.

Polyps in the colon, if large, will be detected by routine barium enema. Small polyps require a very meticulous technique for their demonstration. Since the Malmö technique became widely used it has become clear that small polyps in the colon are common (Fig. 8.2). Pathological studies on necropsy material have confirmed the radiological evidence and have shown that polyps are present in over 20% of patients over the age of 40 years. This raises a difficult problem regarding treatment. At one time it was customary to regard all colonic polyps as potentially malignant. Since radiological studies have shown them to be so common, however, it is difficult to continue to accept this viewpoint. Until comparatively recently, once a colonic polyp had been demonstrated by radiology

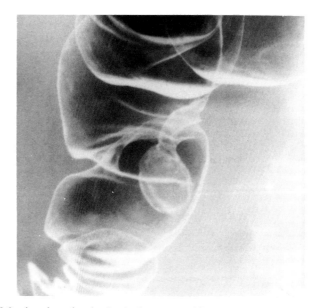

Fig. 8.2 A pedunculated polyp in the erect position.

treatment by surgery was mandatory, but on the present evidence of the high incidence of these polyps a more conservative attitude appears justified. However any polyp larger than 10 mm in diameter, or with a broad base or irregular surface, must be regarded with suspicion. With recent advances in endoscopy many polyps can now be removed without laparotomy.

Chronic amoebic dysentery should be considered in patients with diarrhoea who have returned from, or have lived in, tropical countries or other areas where amoebic dysentery is endemic. In patients with chronic amoebic dysentery there is sometimes a mass or *amoeboma* which superficially may resemble a carcinoma. These may be multiple. Their rapid disappearance with appropriate anti-amoebic therapy will confirm the diagnosis. Amoebic hepatitis if present will also suggest the correct diagnosis.

Chronic colitis can give rise to an irregular shaggy outline of the colonic lumen and occasionally this may occur in a localised form.

Cathartic colon may result from the prolonged use of vegetable cathartics in chronic constipation. The colon becomes atonic and pseudo-strictures, due to inconstant tapering contractions of the colonic wall, may occur. There is loss of haustral pattern first seen on the right side of the colon, which may appear lengthened and widened. The condition may be mistaken for ulcerative colitis, but the strictures are inconstant and the colon wall smooth. These features and an adequate history should enable differentiation to be made.

Ulcerative colitis usually affects a large part of the colon, and in severe cases the entire colon. The mucosa becomes granular and as the disease progresses thickening and fibrosis of the bowel wall occur; in the later stages the colon appears as a narrow tube with little or no haustration (Fig. 8.3). The typical 'hose-pipe' appearance is easy to recognise but it is important to realise that in the early stages ulcerative colitis may be difficult or impossible to diagnose on barium enema. The earliest radiological change is a shaggy or fine serrated appearance of the bowel wall. Later the bowel becomes more ragged and marginal ulceration may become evident. Finally, the thickened fibrosed bowel wall appears as a narrow band. In long-standing cases radiology may be helpful in demonstrating complications such as *pseudo-polyposis* and *carcinoma*. Colonic perforation can be confirmed by the demonstration of free air in the peritoneum.

Crohn's disease can involve the colon and simulate ulcerative colitis. The affected areas are usually less extensive, however, and

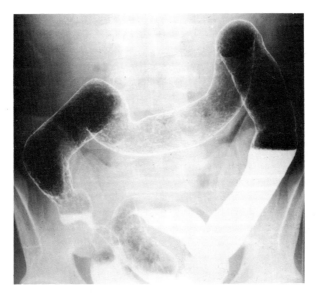

Fig. 8.3 Ulcerative colitis. Fine granularity throughout the colon which is shortened and totally devoid of haustration.

the presence of normal 'skip' areas, ileal lesions, and multiple strictures helps in radiological differentiation. The presence of an external sinus track and of so-called 'rose-thorn' ulcers at the margin of the affected area of colon, are features which should suggest Crohn's disease.

Diverticulosis of the colon is common in middle-aged and elderly patients. Diverticula occur most often in the sigmoid region and appear as multiple flask-like pouches protruding from the bowel lumen. *Diverticulitis* is a common complication. This, again, is usually sigmoid in situation. It gives rise to local spasm and a characteristic 'saw tooth' pattern on barium enema (Fig. 8.4). Clinically these cases may present in a variety of ways and differential diagnosis from neoplasm is often difficult, particularly if an inflammatory mass is present. Sometimes these patients present with chronic diarrhoea and are thought to have a form of colitis.

In most patients the radiological findings are characteristic. Sometimes, however, the inflammatory mass may give rise to intestinal obstruction and, in these cases, not only is the clinical picture difficult to differentiate from obstructive neoplasm but the barium enema may also be confusing. This happens when the enema becomes obstructed by the inflammatory mass and the characteristic features of diverticulitis are not visualised below the obstruction.

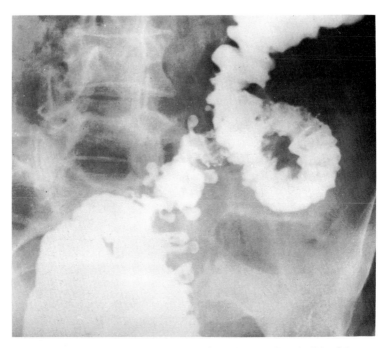

Fig. 8.4 Diverticulosis with some degree of complicating diverticulitis of the sigmoid.

Hirschsprung's disease. The diagnosis is usually made in childhood but the disease may be seen in adults, as may *idiopathic megacolon.* It has been shown that in Hirschsprung's disease there is an aganglionic segment in the sigmoid or distal colon and the colonic dilation is proximal to this abnormal narrowed segment of bowel. The colon above the affected segment is grossly dilated and atonic and barium enema must be performed with caution. The condition is usually suspected clinically and the radiologist should only allow a small quantity of barium to pass through the narrow segment. Otherwise an enormous quantity of barium would be required to fill the dilated colon and would prove difficult to evacuate. The bowel above the stenosed segment is usually so dilated and atonic that a small quantity of barium can easily be moved around it by posturing the patient (Fig. 8.5).

In *idiopathic megacolon* it is not possible to demonstrate a stenosed and aganglionic segment, and the degree of chronic dilatation is usually less marked than in the patient with Hirschsprung's disease.

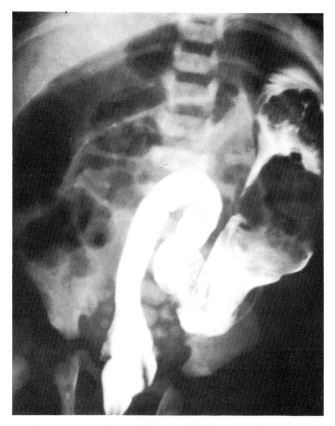

Fig. 8.5 Hirschsprung's disease. There is a fairly long aganglionic segment.

The acute abdomen

Radiology is of considerable assistance in the assessment of patients with an 'acute abdomen'. Investigation is usually by simple X-ray, but in certain circumstances contrast studies may be performed.

Simple X-ray. The occasional snare of the basal pneumonia and pleurisy simulating an acute abdomen can be readily diagnosed by a simple chest X-ray and perforation of the gut shows characteristic radiological appearances of air under the diaphragm.

Perforation. In suspected perforation, whether due to perforating peptic ulcer, ruptured appendix, or to other causes, the cardinal radiological sign is the presence of free air in the peritoneum. This is best demonstrated as layers of air under the diaphragm on an erect film (Fig. 8.6). If the patient is too ill for an erect film, a film can be taken in lateral decubitus with a horizontal X-ray beam. This will demonstrate the intra-peritoneal air in the uppermost flank.

Intestinal obstruction. Radiology is of great help in the assessment of cases of actual or suspected intestinal obstruction. It is the customary routine in most departments to obtain plain films of the abdomen in the supine and erect positions. This is because in acute obstruction it is usual for the bowel to become dilated with air and fluid above the level of an obstruction. In the erect position this shows as horizontal fluid levels in the dilated loops of bowel (Fig. 8.7). These should be assessed in clinical context since there are many other causes of fluid levels in the bowel, e.g. gastro-enteritis, paralytic ileus, uraemia, and congestive cardiac failure.

The appearances in the different areas of the bowel are characteristic. It is usually possible for the radiologist to differentiate on the X-ray film between a high small bowel obstruction, a low small bowel obstruction and a large bowel obstruction. In certain conditions the radiologist may be able to go further and make a specific pathological diagnosis because of characteristic appearances. These may be seen in volvulus of the sigmoid, volvulus of the caecum, intussusception, and in various other conditions.

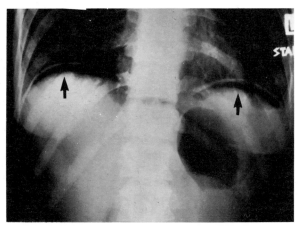

Fig. 8.6   Gas under the diaphragm following perforation of a peptic ulcer. Erect film. Small amounts of air are best seen in a lateral film.

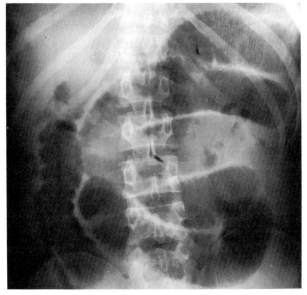

ladder.

(A)

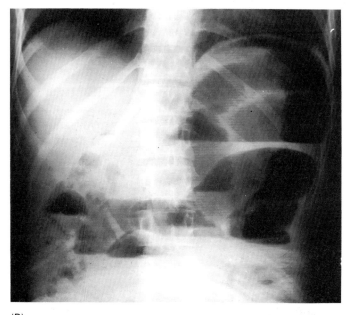

(B)

Fig. 8.7 Small bowel obstruction: (A) supine film showing dilated loops of small bowel in step-ladder pattern; (B) erect film showing air fluid levels.

Volvulus is most commonly seen in the sigmoid colon and usually in elderly patients. The radiological appearances are characteristic and consist of an enormously distended loop of sigmoid projecting up from the pelvis like an inverted letter U. Volvulus of the caecum is less common and is usually associated with an abnormal mesentery attached to the ascending colon. The appearances of volvulus of the caecum are also characteristic and should enable a preoperative diagnosis to be made. The enormously distended caecum is seen below the diaphragm, often in the left hypochondrium or lying centrally.

Subphrenic abscess. Radiology is of great value in proving or disproving a suspected diagnosis of subphrenic abscess. With a subphrenic abscess the diaphragm on the affected side may be elevated and show restricted movement when examined under the fluorescent screen. Sometimes an air fluid level may be demonstrated in a subphrenic abscess when it is examined in the erect position or in lateral decubitus.

Contrast studies. In subacute intestinal obstruction, and occasionally in acute obstruction, contrast studies can prove very helpful. This is particularly so with the barium enema in colonic obstruction. The introduction of Gastrografin also made possible the use of an oral contrast medium in the 'surgical' abdomen, where oral barium is contraindicated.

Colonic obstruction is most commonly due to neoplasm or to diverticulitis. These conditions have already been discussed and barium enema usually permits differentiation. Rarer causes are also seen, such as intussusception and volvulus. *Intussusception* is more commonly seen in children. The barium enema is diagnostic and shows a fine film of barium extending marginally beyond the point of obstruction and between the intussusception and intussuscipiens. It is sometimes possible to reduce the intussusception by means of the diagnostic barium enema. Intussusception in adults is usually associated with the presence of a polypoid tumour in the colon.

Gastrografin, which is a water-soluble organic iodide preparation, can be given by mouth to patients with an acute abdomen in whom the use of barium is contraindicated. Thus it can even be administered to a patient with a suspected perforation, or an intestinal leak (either spontaneous or following surgery) to demonstrate the site of the leak (Fig. 8.8). Should the Gastrografin leak from the bowel it is readily reabsorbed from the peritoneum or retroperitoneal tissues.

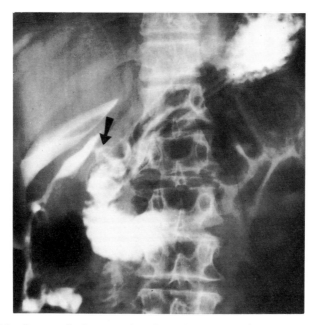

Fig. 8.8   Gastrografin demonstration of a perforated ulcer (↓). Note spread of contrast into peritoneum.

Miscellaneous abdominal conditions

Foreign bodies. A recurring problem to the radiologist is the swallowed foreign body or the suspected swallowed foreign body. When a child has swallowed a small coin such as a penny, or when the foreign body is seen to have no sharp edges, repeated X-rays are not necessary. The vast majority of swallowed foreign bodies seen in children or adults are passed without any trouble whatsoever. Only if the foreign body is large relative to the gut lumen, or has sharp points, e.g. an open safety-pin, are such measures really necessary, and only if the foreign body has become impacted or appears on serial X-ray to be fixed in one part of the gut is there any cause for alarm. It is surprising, however, how rarely actual perforation of the gut or obstruction by a swallowed foreign body occurs. A conservative policy of observation of the patient rather than immediate surgery will often prevent an unnecessary laparotomy.

Steroids and the alimentary tract. Cortisone is so widely prescribed at the present day that it behoves the student to be aware of possible alimentary complications of cortisone therapy. Thus *duodenal ulceration* may occur, and a duodenal ulcer may even perforate with the symptoms masked by cortisone. The possibility of duodenal ulceration or of silent perforations should therefore be borne in mind in the case of any patient who is on prolonged steroid therapy.

9. The biliary tract, liver and pancreas

THE BILIARY TRACT

A wide variety of techniques for imaging the biliary system now exists. These include:

1. Simple X-rays
2. Oral cholecystography
3. Intravenous cholangiography
4. Operative and postoperative cholangiography
5. Percutaneous transhepatic cholangiography (PTC)
6. Endoscopic retrograde cholangio-pancreatography (ERCP)
7. Ultrasound
8. Isotope scanning
9. Computed tomography (CT)
10. Magnetic resonance imaging (MRI).

In many cases the clinical features point clearly to disease of the biliary tract. Thus with clinical symptoms of biliary colic or with obstructive jaundice there is little doubt as to the system to be investigated. In other cases, however, the symptoms are more vague, and may merely consist of dyspepsia or other indefinite abdominal symptoms. Thus it is not uncommon for the radiologist to be asked to investigate the gastro-intestinal tract before suspicion is finally centred on the biliary tract. This problem of vague dyspepsia (? peptic ulcer ? biliary) is so common that at some centres the investigation of both the biliary tract and the stomach and duodenum are carried out at the same examination. This is done by performing an oral cholecystogram in a routine manner, and when the patient attends for X-ray of the contrast-filled gall-bladder a barium meal is performed immediately. Most radiologists, however, prefer to perform the two investigations at separate sessions.

Simple X-rays of the biliary tract

Opaque gall-stones will be readily shown. These vary in type (Fig. 9.1). They may be large laminated structures, which are usually solitary or few in number. On the other hand small calculi may be multiple and numerous. An opaque stone in the cystic or

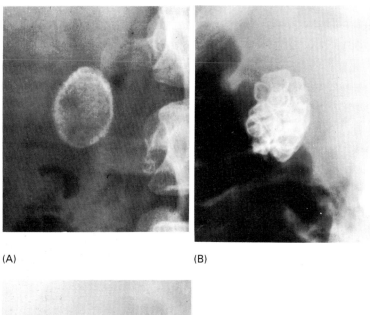

(A)   (B)

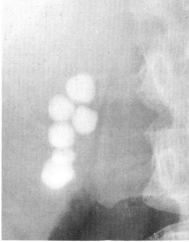

(C)

Fig. 9.1 Different types of biliary calculi in the gall-bladder. (A) Large and (B) small mixed stones with translucent cholesterol centres, (C) infective stones with dense calcium carbonate deposits.

common bile duct can be diagnosed by its position relative to the normal gall-bladder. This is easy if there are also opaque stones in the gall-bladder.

Non-opaque gall-stones, for instance large cholesterol stones, will not be diagnosed by plain X-rays and will require contrast studies (Fig. 9.2), or ultrasound for their demonstration. Multiple minute calculi may form a sediment in the gall-bladder giving rise to so-called 'milky bile'. This will outline the whole gall-bladder in the supine patient and will sediment to form a horizontal level in the gall-bladder in the erect film.

Occasionally calcification may occur in the wall of a chronically diseased gall-bladder – the so-called 'porcelain gall-bladder' outlined at simple X-ray (Fig. 9.3).

Gas in the biliary tract, usually in the hepatic ducts, is only occasionally noted at plain X-ray (Fig. 9.4). This implies either a

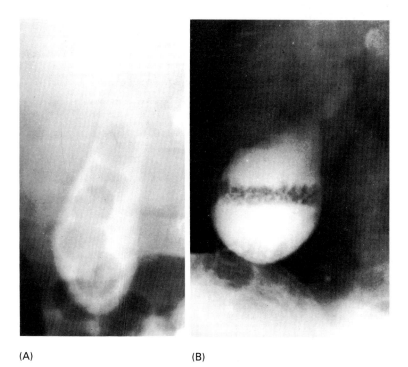

(A) (B)

Fig. 9.2 (A) Large non-opaque cholesterol calculi visible in a contrast-filled gall-bladder. (B) Multiple small non-opaque calculi shown floating as a horizontal level in an erect film.

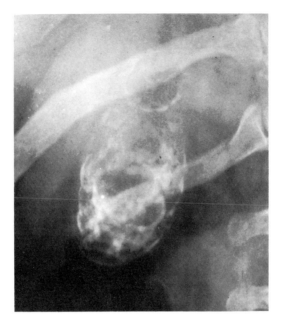

Fig. 9.3   Calcification of the gall-bladder wall.

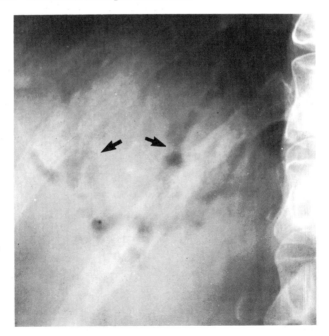

Fig. 9.4   Gas in the biliary ducts.

fistula between the bowel and the biliary tract, or an incompetent sphincter of Oddi. The latter condition may be seen following passage of a large calculus or following operative intervention and exploration.

It is important to remember that both oral and intravenous cholecystography are unlikely to be successful in the presence of *obstructive jaundice*. This is because with biliary obstruction the excretion of contrast from the liver is impaired.

Oral cholecystography

The technique for oral cholecystography requires the patient to take the contrast medium by mouth the evening before the examination. He remains on a fat-free diet until he attends for X-ray examination some 16 hours later. At this stage the gall-bladder is usually well filled with contrast. Once this has been verified the patient is given a fatty meal.

This will induce contraction of the gall-bladder within 10 to 30 minutes. Further films are then taken which show the normal gall-bladder to have contracted well, and may demonstrate the contrast-filled cystic and common bile ducts, and the entry of contrast into the duodenum (Fig. 9.5).

Non-opaque calculi lying in the gall-bladder will be demonstrated as filling defects within the contrast-filled lumen (Fig. 9.2). Failure of the gall-bladder to opacify on oral cholecystography is very suggestive of gall-bladder disease, or of obstruction of the cystic ducts by calculus, but is not conclusive. This is because excretion by the liver depends on absorption of the contrast medium by the alimentary tract. A proportion of patients have diarrhoea following ingestion of the oral medium and the amount absorbed from the gut is therefore unpredictable. In patients with severe liver disease or with biliary obstruction excretion from the liver may also be impaired.

Tumours of the gall-bladder. Carcinoma of the gall-bladder is diagnosed on clinical grounds and radiology, including cholecystography, has proved of no assistance in arriving at a diagnosis though ultrasound, CT and MRI may be helpful, particularly in staging. Benign tumours of the gall-bladder are occasionally seen and these can be diagnosed by cholecystography. *Papillomas* are seen as small translucent defects at the lateral margin of the gall-bladder, whilst *adenomas* are seen as small translucent defects attached to the fundus. Carcinoma of the common bile duct usually presents with

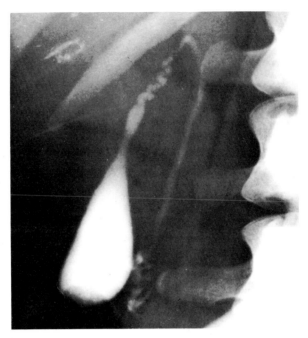

Fig. 9.5   Contracted gall-bladder after a fatty meal with filling of the cystic and common bile ducts and entry of contrast into the duodenum.

obstructive jaundice and is diagnosed when direct cholangiography or ultrasound shows a typical obstruction to the dilated common duct.

Intravenous cholangiography

This was widely practised at one time but toxic reactions were not infrequent and it has been rendered obsolete by ultrasound and CT.

Ultrasound

This is now widely used as the preliminary examination in suspected gall-bladder or biliary tract disease and has the added advantage that the liver and pancreas can be assessed at the same examination. It is highly accurate in the diagnosis of gallstones including the non-opaque stones not visible at simple radiography.

Gallstones characteristically produce high density echoes and cast acoustic shadows appearing as dark bands (Fig. 9.6).

Ultrasound will also demonstrate dilated intrahepatic bile ducts or a dilated common bile duct and thus will help to differentiate obstructive from non-obstructive jaundice (Fig. 9.7).

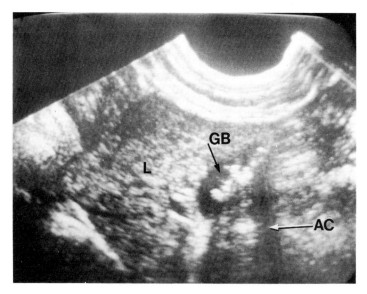

Fig. 9.6   Gallstones. Note the acoustic shadows causing dark bands behind the gall-bladder. L = liver. GB = gall-bladder with stones. AC = acoustic shadows.

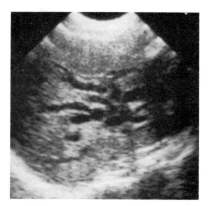

Fig. 9.7   Dilated intrahepatic bile ducts shown by ultrasound.

Isotope scanning

^{99}Tc^m HIDA (a derivative of iminodiacetic acid (IDA)) is a drug which is concentrated by the hepatocytes and excreted in the bile. Serial gamma camera pictures taken at 10 minute intervals after administration show the normal gall-bladder and biliary tract at 30 min and drainage into the gut at 60 min (Fig. 9.8). In biliary obstruction there is no evidence of gut activity even on delayed films at 24 h. HIDA is also a most valuable screening test for acute cholecystitis when the gall-bladder will fail to fill despite gut activity. Similar appearances are seen if the cystic duct or Hartmann's pouch are obstructed by calculi.

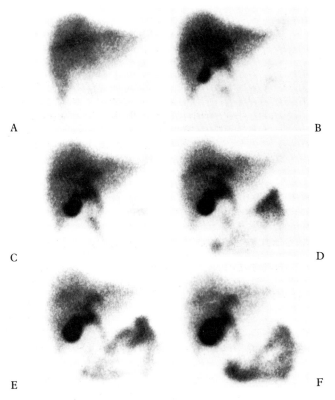

A   B

C   D

E   F

Fig. 9.8 Biliary scan (^{99}Tc^m HIDA). Serial films. (A) 5 minutes, (B) 10 minutes. (C) 15 minutes.(D) 20 minutes. (E) 25 minutes and (F) 30 minutes after injection. Contrast is seen in the bowel at 20 minutes. Note concentration in gall-bladder from B onward.

Operative and postoperative cholangiography

It is well known that in calculous biliary disease cholecystectomy alone will leave a proportion of patients with residual stones in the biliary ducts. On the other hand exploration of the ducts adds considerably to the risk of the operation and may miss stones which are free to move about in the ducts or are of soft consistency ('putty stones'). Many surgeons now perform operative cholangiography as a routine at operations for biliary stones. A small tube is inserted into the cystic duct and the bile ducts are filled with contrast medium. Films are obtained and examined during the operation and should demonstrate most removable calculi in the ducts.

Operative cholangiography, if skilfully performed, adds little to the operative time and will ensure against leaving stones in the duct which may require a second operation. The best results are obtained when there is direct co-operation between surgeon and radiologist and apparatus permitting serial film is used. The possibility of artefact due to gas bubbles must be borne in mind and guarded against.

Postoperative cholangiography is carried out in the immediate postoperative period by injecting the T-tube drain in the common bile duct with contrast medium (Fig. 9.9). This method will also show residual calculi which have been missed at operation. These can be removed with a catheter snare passed through the T-tube tract under image intensifier control.

Operative and postoperative cholangiography are also useful for demonstrating strictures of the common bile duct and in assessing neoplastic obstruction.

Percutaneous transhepatic cholangiography (PTC)

The main indication for percutaneous cholangiography is in the assessment of obstructive jaundice. If the bile ducts are grossly dilated there is usually little difficulty in puncturing a dilated duct percutaneously. Once a hepatic duct has been entered, bile can be aspirated and contrast medium injected (Fig. 9.10). This enables the site of obstruction to be demonstrated and its characteristics to be studied. A diagnosis of obstructive carcinoma, stone or stricture, can then be confirmed. The puncture is made percutaneously from the right flank using a fine needle and after preliminary infiltration of the skin and subcutaneous tissues with a local anaesthetic. The prothrombin time should not be more than three seconds prolonged.

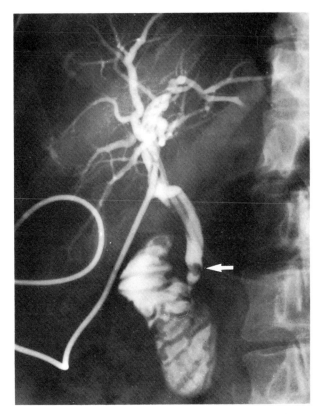

Fig. 9.9 Postoperative T-tube cholangiogram showing free entry of contrast into the duodenum despite a residual non-opaque calculus at the lower end of the common hepatic duct (←).

Percutaneous biliary drainage can also be performed via a special needle catheter assembly. After a preliminary fine needle percutaneous cholangiogram one of the main ducts is catheterised percutaneously under screen control. The obstructed ducts can then be drained with an indwelling catheter as a palliative measure or as a preliminary to surgery. A further refinement of this technique is the percutaneous insertion of a drain through a stenosis or obstructed common duct into the duodenum.

Endoscopic retrograde cholangiography (ERC) is a technique which is being increasingly used and has largely replaced PTC. The technique is essentially similar to ERCP described below, and can be performed safely even when the prothrombin time is significantly prolonged.

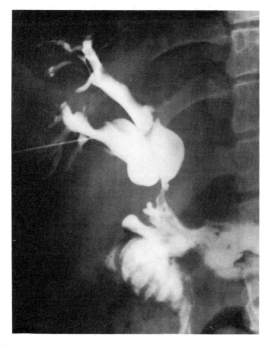

Fig. 9.10 Percutaneous cholangiogram in a patient with obstructive jaundice. This patient had a congenital choledochal cyst treated by anastomosis to the gut. This was followed years later by an anastomotic stricture.

Endoscopic retrograde cholangio-pancreatography (ERCP)

Under radiological control the ampulla of Vater is cannulated and the common bile duct or pancreatic duct can be entered. Contrast medium can then be injected and the biliary or pancreatic ducts can be shown (Fig. 9.11). Biliary obstruction due to stone or neoplasm can be visualised, or alternatively a normal biliary tree may be shown. In skilled hands this is probably the method of choice for the investigation of obstructive jaundice. It is also of great value in the investigation of pancreatic disease. Not only can the pancreatic duct be injected and shown to be normal, abnormal, or obstructed but pancreatic juice can be directly collected and analysed.

For this examination the patient is usually fasting and lightly sedated. A side viewing duodenoscope or other fibre-scope is passed to the duodenum. The ampulla of Vater is identified and a small Teflon catheter is passed from the endoscope into the apex of the papilla under visual control.

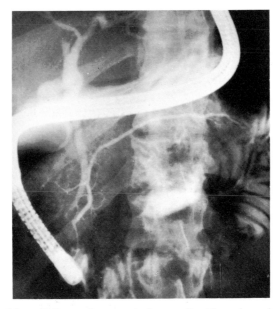

Fig. 9.11 Normal biliary and pancreatic ducts outlined by endoscopic retrograde cholangio-pancreatography.

THE LIVER

The main indications for investigation of the liver by imaging are the diagnosis or exclusion of tumours, primary and secondary, of cysts and of inflammatory lesions. Other indications are the investigation of hepatomegaly, of cirrhosis and of portal hypertension.

The techniques available include:

1. Simple X-ray
2. Ultrasound
3. CT
4. Isotope scanning
5. MRI
6. Hepatic angiography
7. Splenic and arterial portography.

Simple X-ray provides little information apart from confirming enlargement of the liver and showing the occasional calcified lesion such as some hydatid cysts.

Ultrasound

Ultrasound is widely used in the investigation of the liver and biliary systems (Fig. 9.12). Within the liver cysts, abscesses, haematomas and neoplasms both primary and secondary are readily identified. Tumours usually show as rounded areas with diminished echoes (Fig. 9.13), though occasionally, as with some colonic secondaries, high intensity echoes are seen (Fig. 9.14). Cysts are completely transonic (Fig. 9.15). As already noted above dilated bile ducts are identifiable and are characteristic of obstructive jaundice. The gall-bladder and gallstones are also readily shown.

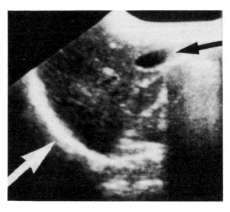

Fig. 9.12 Normal liver and gall-bladder. Longitudinal scan. The gall-bladder appears as a well-defined oval transonic organ (black arrow) anteriorly. The diaphragm produces the curved line (white arrow) posteriorly.

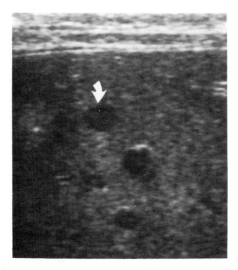

Fig. 9.13 Multiple small metastases (arrow = halo).

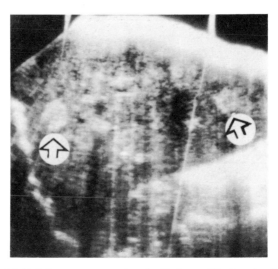

Fig. 9.14   Multiple liver metastases. Longitudinal scan. The liver is enlarged and there are multiple areas of high echogenicity (arrows), scattered through it indicating metastases. Primary tumour in large bowel.

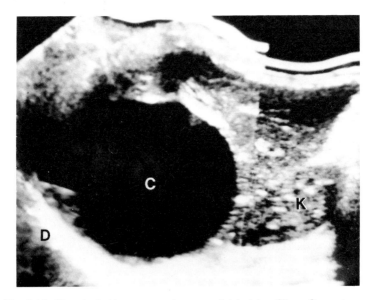

Fig. 9.15   Huge hydatid cyst occupying most of right lobe of liver. C = cyst. K = kidney. D = diaphragm.

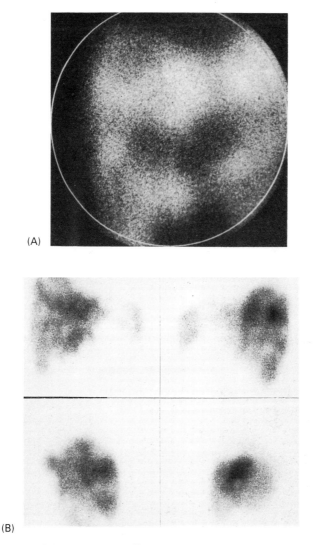

(A)

(B)

Fig. 9.16 (A) Liver metastases. $^{99}Tc^m$-S colloid scan. Anterior projection. The liver is large and contains many defects caused by metastases. (B) $^{99}Tc^m$ colloid scan of liver. Multiple metastases from carcinoma of the colon showing numerous areas of low altenuation.

Isotope scanning

Following an intravenous injection of $^{99}Tc^m$ colloid the normal liver substance takes up the isotope uniformly and is easily imaged. Most pathological lesions – tumours, cysts, abscesses and haematomas – do not take up the compound and appear as filling defects in the opacified liver (Fig. 9.16). Provided the individual lesions are larger than 2 cm in diameter most tumours are clearly seen, though they cannot be differentiated from benign lesions purely on the scan. All scans must be interpreted in the light of the clinical features, though multiple defects are always suggestive of metastases.

CT scanning

CT shows the liver in axial sections with high resolution. Primary and secondary neoplasms can be demonstrated and differentiated from cysts (Figs 9.17 and 9.18). Adjacent organs are also shown on the scans including abdominal nodes thus making CT invaluable in the staging of tumours.

Contrast enhancement following intravenous injection is frequently undertaken to highlight focal lesions. Dynamic scans involving rapid serial images after contrast injection may assist in diagnosing vascular lesions such as haemangiomas and some tumours.

MRI

MRI is similar to CT in the accuracy of showing focal lesions in the liver. It has the advantage of easy imaging in the coronal and sagittal planes but is still relatively more costly than CT.

Angiography

Hepatic angiography is performed by percutaneous transfemoral catheterisation of the coeliac axis or superselective catheterisation of the hepatic artery followed by injection of a bolus of contrast medium. The technique was once widely used for the diagnosis of tumours (Fig. 9.19), but has been superseded for this purpose by the less invasive techniques just described. Angiomas, aneurysms and other vascular lesions can be precisely defined by angiography and the technique is also used for the transcatheter embolisation

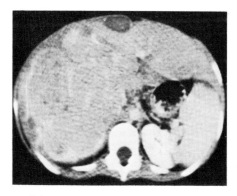

Fig. 9.17 Hepatocellular carcinoma. Most of the right lobe of liver replaced by tumour with rim enhancement after contrast.

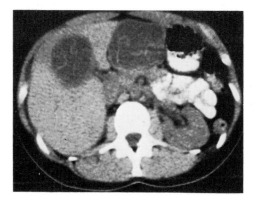

Fig. 9.18 Hydatid disease. Large hydatid cysts in right and left lobe of liver together with daughter cysts.

of vascular lesions as well as tumours. It is also utilised for the treatment of tumours by local chemotherapy drug infusion.

Portography, or imaging of the portal system, can be achieved in several ways:

1. *Splenic portography*. This was once widely performed by direct injection of the spleen from a percutaneous needle puncture in the flank (Fig. 9.20), but has been renderd obsolete by other techniques.

2. *Arterial portography* is achieved by delayed filming after percutaneous catheterisation and injection of the splenic and superior mesenteric arteries allowing time for the contrast bolus to

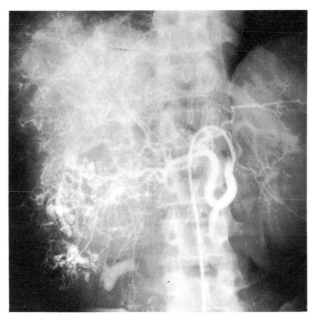

Fig. 9.19 Selective hepatic arteriogram. A large vascular tumour is shown in the lower part of the right lobe of the liver. Histology: primary hepatoma.

pass through the vascular bed and drain into the splenic or superior mesenteric veins and on into the portal vein. DSA enhances the quality of the resultant images of the portal circulation.

3. *Transhepatic portography* is achieved by passing a needle catheter assembly through the liver from the right flank and siting the tip in a portal branch using image intensifier screening control. The catheter can then be guided to different sites in the portal system. Normal blood clotting factors are essential and the track in the liver is embolised with gelfoam on withdrawal of the catheter. This route is used for demonstration and embolisation of varices (Fig. 9.21) and for venous sampling.

Choice of examination in biliary and liver disease

The large battery of tests now available can give rise to over-investigation and careful clinical judgement is required as to which tests should be used in particular circumstances. To some extent this will be conditioned by local availability of apparatus such as CT

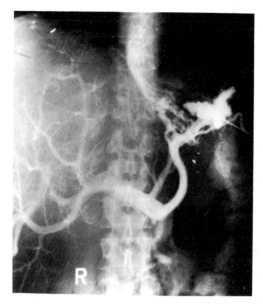

Fig. 9.20 Percutaneous splenic phlebogram. The splenic and portal veins are patent and there is good filling of the intra-hepatic branches of the portal vein. There is reflux filling of the oesophageal varices.

or ultrasound, and local skills and expertise. However, where all techniques are available, primary investigation should be by non-invasive techniques. The more invasive methods such as percutaneous cholangiography and angiography should be reserved for specific indications.

Suspected liver masses (tumours, primary or secondary; cysts and abscesses) should be examined in the first place by isotope scanning or ultrasound. Both these methods will usually demonstrate liver masses quite well. Ultrasound has the advantage that it will differentiate cysts and abscesses from solid masses. CT and MRI will also perform this function but are more expensive investigations and CT involves radiation. They are used for more precise diagnosis; as a prelude to surgery; and for tumour staging.

In suspected obstructive jaundice ultrasound is the primary investigation of choice, though biliary isotope scanning will show moderately dilated ducts, as will CT. Transhepatic cholangiography or ERCP may be required to define the point of obstruction, and percutaneous biliary drainage may be used in treatment.

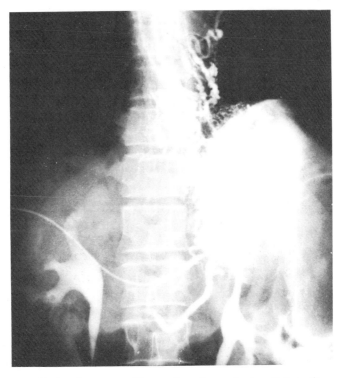

Fig. 9.21 Varices demonstrated by transhepatic portal vein catheterization.

THE PANCREAS

Diseases of the pancreas demonstrable by imaging include inflammatory lesions (acute and chronic pancreatitis), cysts and tumours.

Simple X-ray will occasionally show extensive nodules of calcification in the pancreas associated with chronic pancreatitis but is otherwise of little help.

Barium studies will show distortion of the duodenal loop by masses in the head of the pancreas and large pancreatic masses or cysts may displace the stomach.

Ultrasound. The normal pancreas may be partly obscured by bowel gas but when well seen appears as a 1 to 3 cm diameter band arching over the aorta at the level of the superior mesenteric artery and of slightly higher echogenicity than normal liver. In acute pancreatitis the whole organ is enlarged and oedematous appearing more transonic than normal. Abscesses and cysts appear as well defined rounded transonic areas (Fig. 9.22). Tumours appear as local masses enlarging the pancreas.

CT is now the method most widely used for the demonstration of pancreatic morphology (Fig. 9.23). The pancreas and its relationships to adjacent organs are clearly identified; cysts and mass lesions greater than 2 cm in diameter are easily identified (Fig. 9.24). Small tumours such as islet cell adenomas are more difficult to diagnose. Acute pancreatitis may be clearly demonstrated at CT as diffuse swelling and oedema of the whole organ, though some cases,

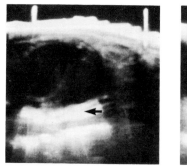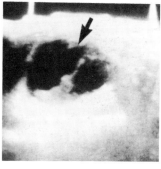

(A)   (B)

Fig. 9.22 Pancreatic pseudocyst. Longitudinal scans. (A) Low power. The huge pseudocyst is shown as a large transonic mass in front of the aorta and superior mesenteric artery (arrow). (B) High power. The outline of the cyst is better seen (arrow) and a septum and echoes are shown within it.

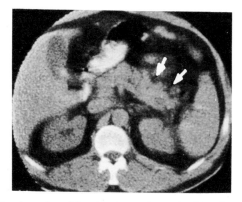

Fig. 9.23 Normal pancreas. Note lobulation of outline in obese patient. Arrows point to tail. (L + 10 W200).

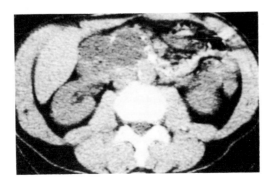

Fig. 9.24 Chronic pancreatitis. Paraductal cysts deform and enlarge the pancreatic head which appears as a low density area anterior to the right kidney, inferior vena cava, and aorta. Note calcification (L0 W200).

particularly in the first 24 hours, will not show diagnostic appearances. Dilatation and irregularity of the main pancreatic duct can also be seen at CT.

MRI can also show the pancreas well but has no advantages over CT, which is much cheaper and more readily available.

ERCP is the method of choice for demonstrating the pancreatic duct (Fig. 9.11) and its obstruction or stenosis by calculi or tumour. The bile ducts can be demonstrated at the same time and a variety of diagnostic and therapeutic procedures performed. These include:

1. Stone extraction from pancreatic and bile ducts
2. Sphincterotomy
3. Biopsy of ampulla
4. Cytology of pancreatic juice or brushings
5. Balloon dilatation of benign strictures
6. Biliary stent insertion
7. Pancreatic cyst drainage.

Choice of examination

CT is probably the best method for speedy demonstration of the pancreas. The normal pancreas is usually well shown as are masses and cysts. Small tumours whether carcinomas or islet cell adenomas are more difficult to define. Ultrasound in skilled hands is almost as reliable, but is to some extent operator dependent.

Isotope scanning is less reliable than CT or ultrasound and is no longer used for pancreatic lesions. Neither CT nor ultrasound will differentiate an inflammatory pancreatic mass from a tumorous lesion. However, *fine needle biopsy* guided by CT or ultrasound will permit a definitive diagnosis (Fig. 13.3).

10. The urinary tract and the adrenals

The following radiological and imaging methods are available for the investigation of the urinary tract:

1. Simple radiology
2. Intravenous urography
3. Retrograde pyelography
4. Antegrade pyelography
5. Renal angiography
6. Cystography, cysto-urethrography and dynamic bladder studies
7. Urethrography
8. Cyst puncture
9. Ultrasound
10. Computed tomography
11. Isotope imaging and renography
12. MRI.

Plain X-rays

Plain X-rays of the renal tract are taken as a routine before most kidney investigations. Good-quality films will often show the renal outlines quite clearly, and gross enlargement of the kidney by hydronephrosis or tumour may be readily recognised. Similarly, gross shrinkage of the kidney from chronic pyelonephritis or from renal ischaemia may be diagnosed.

Calcification in the renal areas is most commonly due to renal *calculi* in the calyces or renal pelvis. *Nephrocalcinosis,* or calcification within the renal substance, is much less common, and is seen in such rare conditions as *hyperparathyroidism, renal tubular acidosis,* and *medullary sponge kidney.* Calcification may also be observed in the kidney in *renal tuberculosis,* and occasionally in *renal tumours.*

Plain X-rays will also demonstrate opaque *calculi* in the ureter and in the bladder (Fig. 10.1). Calcification in the bladder wall and

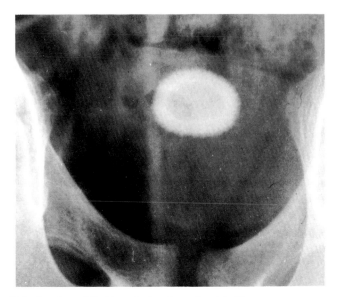

Fig. 10.1 Laminated bladder calculus shown by plain X-ray.

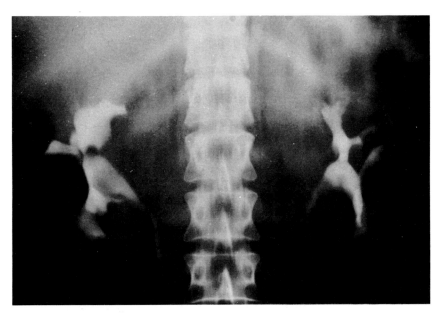

Fig. 10.2 Polycystic kidneys. Note the bilateral splaying and deformity of the minor calyces and large size of the kidneys.

ureter is seen in *schistosomiasis*. Very rarely calcification may be detected in bladder tumours due to encrustations on the surface of a tumour.

Intravenous urogaphy (IVU)

Provided that the kidney is functioning and the blood urea is not too high intravenous urography will demonstrate most lesions affecting the normal anatomy of the renal drainage system.

Congenital anomalies, such as double pelves and ureters, or duplex and horse-shoe kidneys, can be diagnosed with certainty. *Polycystic kidneys* can also be identified unless renal failure has supervened. In a typical case both kidneys are enlarged, and there are multiple calyceal deformities (Fig. 10.2).

Local distortion of the renal calyces by a kidney mass is often seen on urography (Fig. 10.3). In many of these cases it is impossible to differentiate between *hypernephroma* and a *simple cyst* from the

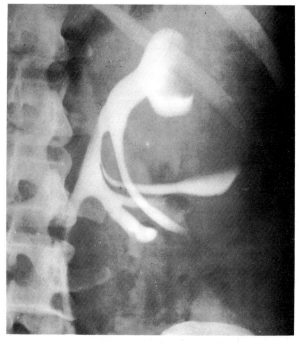

Fig. 10.3 Hypernephroma producing bizarre deformity and stretching of the renal calyces.

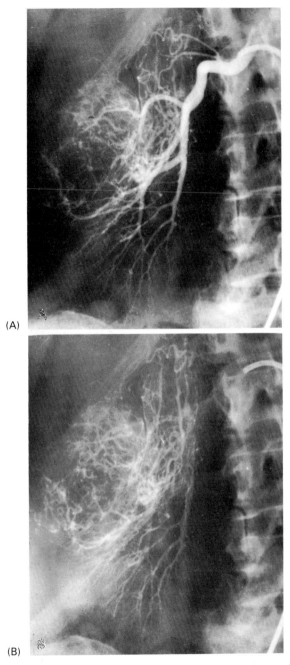

(A)

(B)

Fig. 10.4   (A and B) Renal angiography in a case of renal carcinoma showing pathological vessels.

pyelogram. In such cases imaging by ultrasound will provide a definitive answer and is the next investigation of choice. CT will also differentiate renal tumour from cyst. If a cyst is demonstrated the diagnosis can be confirmed by percutaneous cyst puncture, and the cyst can then be emptied by aspiration. If a tumour is diagnosed or suggested by ultrasound the diagnosis can be confirmed by CT. This will also help staging and show whether the renal vein is involved. Arteriography will also confirm the diagnosis of tumour (Fig. 10.4), but is now little used except where embolisation is being considered.

Calyceal excavation due to *tuberculosis* can also be identified on intravenous urography, as can the characteristic small pericalyceal cysts of *medullary sponge kidney*. Hydronephrosis may be demonstrated and the site of obstruction will be shown (Fig. 10.5). In *chronic pyelonephritis* irregular shrinkage of the renal cortex and dilatation of the calyces can be recognised.

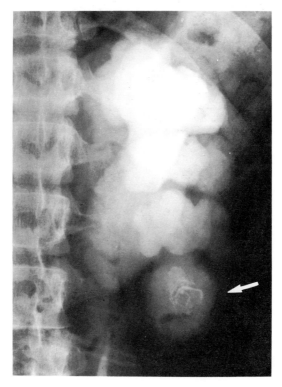

Fig. 10.5 Hydronephrosis with a calculus in the dilated lower calyx (←).

Opaque or suspected non-opaque *renal calculi* may be further investigated by intravenous urography. The relationship of an opaque renal calculus or of a suspected renal calculus to the ureter, pelvis or calyces is clearly demonstrated (Fig. 10.5). Non-opaque calculi are shown as filling defects which may be obstructing the renal drainage system and causing hydroureter and hydronephrosis proximal to the level of the obstruction.

The bladder is also well shown at intravenous urography. *Bladder tumours* whether papillomatous or carcinomatous can be demonstrated (Fig. 10.6) though such tumours may be better visualised by cystography.

Prostatic lesions with bladder-neck obstruction are often assessed by intravenous urography. The *enlarged prostate* may show as a large rounded filling defect at the neck of the bladder. The bladder itself may show trabeculation and thickening of its wall and there may also be evidence of back pressure on the kidneys. *Diverticula* of the bladder, which are more frequent in the elderly patient with bladder-neck obstruction, can also be seen. In prostatic problems it is vital to obtain a film of the bladder after micturition, as the amount of residual urine gives a good index of the degree of obstruction.

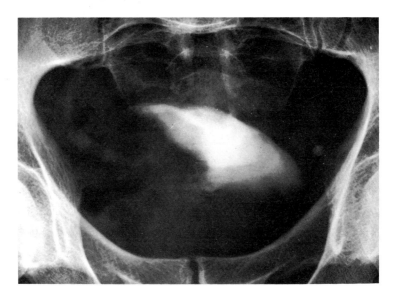

Fig. 10.6 Large filling defect deforming the bladder and due to neoplasm.

Hypertension of possible renal origin is also investigated by intravenous urography in the first instance. This will demonstrate unilateral or bilateral hydronephrosis and will direct attention to the unilateral non-functioning kidney or to polycystic kidneys. Intravenous urography may also show a characteristic pattern in hypertensive patients in whom the cause is unilateral ischaemia of a kidney. In these patients, in whom the usual causative lesion is an atheromatous plaque stenosing the main renal artery (Fig. 10.7), the ischaemic kidney is small and shows increased density of contrast in the pelvis and calyces as the examination proceeds. This is because there is a greater percentage of water resorption on the affected side than on the normal side.

Retrograde pyelography

Retrograde pyelography is performed after cystoscopy and the insertion of a radiopaque ureteric catheter by the surgeon. A small quantity of sterile contrast medium is injected up the catheter to outline the renal tract and appropriate films are taken. The retrograde pyelogram was once used as a method of clearly defining

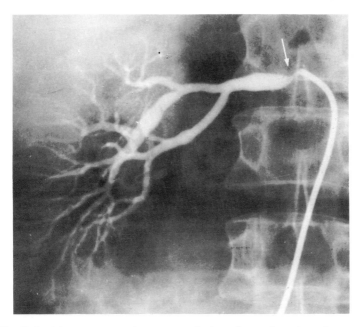

Fig. 10.7 Atheromatous renal artery stenosis shown by renal arteriography.

the anatomy of the renal drainage system in the patient with a non-functioning kidney or with a poorly functioning kidney when intravenous pyelography had failed to provide adequate visualisation. It is less widely practised today than in the past because the modern intravenous contrast media with the use of high dosage and delayed films often provide diagnostic results where the older contrast media might have been unsuccessful, and also because cases of suspected tumour or cyst are now usually investigated by ultrasound or other methods mentioned above.

Retrograde pyelography is still sometimes used to confirm or disprove the relationship of a suspected small calculus to the ureter. It is also sometimes used to help dislodge a ureteric calculus and 'oil' it down the ureter.

Antegrade pyelography (percutaneous nephrostomy)

Percutaneous antegrade pyelography is a useful method of demonstrating the renal calyces, pelvis and ureter in cases of suspected urinary tract obstruction where the intravenous method has been unsuccessful or inconclusive. Unlike retrograde urography it does not require GA and it has a lower incidence of urinary tract infection. It is also useful in infants and children where cystoscopy is difficult or impossible.

A dilated renal calyx is punctured percutaneously from the lumbar region using a fine needle, and contrast medium is injected. The technique can also be used to insert a catheter and provide temporary drainage. The catheter tract can also be used for a percutaneous approach to renal calculi and for stent insertions.

Renal angiography

An opaque catheter is passed percutaneously into the aorta and its preshaped tip is screened into the renal artery origin with the aid of an image intensifier. The whole renal circulation can be beautifully demonstrated using only a small quantity of low-concentration contrast medium.

The renal angiogram in the past provided a method of making a preoperative differential diagnosis in the difficult cases in which a mass had been demonstrated in the kidney but it was uncertain whether this was due to a tumour or cyst. The typical hypernephroma shows excessive vascularity with pathological vessels throughout the tumour area (Fig. 10.4). The typical cyst appears as a large rounded defect in the angiogram. The method was highly accurate in differentiating between tumours and cysts though occasionally a non-vascular tumour was encountered which gave rise to difficulty. As noted above ultrasound or CT now provide simpler methods of confirming the diagnosis of renal cyst or tumour.

Renal angiography has also been widely used for the embolisation of vascular tumours and for the investigation of renal hypertension. A small proportion of patients with hypertension are suffering from renal ischaemia with secondary hypertension. The usual cause is an atheromatous narrowing of the origin of a renal artery (Fig. 10.7). Other less common causes of renal artery stenosis include a peculiar condition occurring mainly in female patients and termed *fibromuscular hyperplasia* of the renal artery (Fig. 10.8). Renal artery stenosis shown by angiography can now be treated by percutaneous dilatation with a Gruntzig balloon catheter.

Cystography

Cystography is performed after passage of a catheter into the

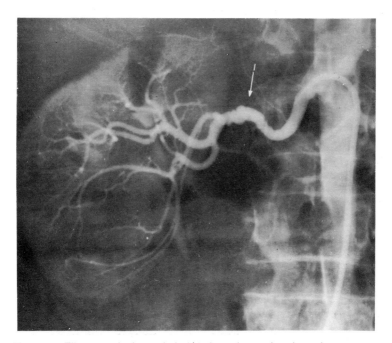

Fig. 10.8 Fibromuscular hyperplasia (↓) shown by renal angiography.

bladder and injection of contrast medium. The method is useful for outlining tumours of the bladder when intravenous urography has been unsuccessful or equivocal. Ultrasound can also be used to demonstrate bladder tumours and CT or MRI enables such tumours to be assessed and staged.

Attention has been drawn to the frequent occurrence of *vesico-ureteric reflux* and to the importance of this condition in the pathogenesis of chronic pyelonephritis. It is claimed that vesico-ureteric reflux is present in a high proportion of patients with chronic pyelonephritis, and that it may be an important etiological factor. Reflux is best demonstrated by performing a *micturating cystogram*, though it may occur spontaneously when the bladder is well filled (Fig. 10.9). As the patient micturates, reflux up the ureters may be seen as the bladder contracts.

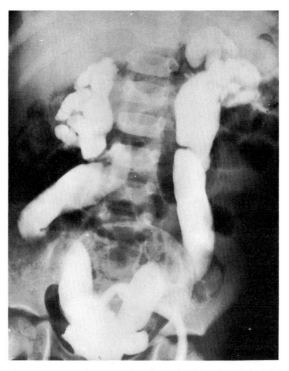

Fig. 10.9 Spontaneous vesico-ureteric reflux after injection of the bladder through an indwelling catheter. There is already gross hydro-ureter and hydronephrosis. (Urethral obstruction in a child due to congenital valves.)

Cysto-urethrography

This examination is used for the investigation of bladder-neck obstruction in males, the various forms of bladder-neck disturbance seen in postpartum females, and other disorders of the peripheral control of micturition.

The technique is to fill the bladder via a catheter which is then removed. The act of micturition is observed on the screen and films of the bladder-neck and urethra taken during micturition. As already noted, vesico-ureteric reflux may be observed during this procedure and is an important finding. The procedure is performed with the aid of an image intensifier. This has the added advantage that it is possible to take a cine film or videorecord of the act of micturition. This can then be played back and details observed at leisure.

Dynamic bladder studies are indicated in more complicated bladder problems with incontinence, frequency, disorders of storage function and voiding, neuropathic bladder and postoperative disturbed function. Various physiological measurements are superimposed upon a video image of the bladder and urethra during filling and voiding. These measurements are the *abdominal* and *bladder pressures* (recorded by rectal and bladder transducers respectively), the detrusor or *intrinsic bladder pressure* (the recorded bladder pressure minus the abdominal pressure) and the *urine flow rate*. Analysis of these synchronous recordings permits improved evaluation of the mechanisms of the bladder dysfunction.

Urethrography

Urethrography in the male is usually performed by injection of a viscous contrast medium which provides excellent contrast throughout the urethra. The contrast medium is injected after insertion of a tight-fitting nozzle into the meatus and the whole of the urethra is outlined. Obstruction by a stricture can then be localised, and in the case of prostatic problems the prostatic urethra can be carefully studied.

Cyst puncture

Renal cysts can be punctured percutaneously from the lumbar region. This is best done under ultrasound control when the point of puncture and the depth and size of the cyst can be assessed.

The straw-coloured fluid they contain is aspirated. Once the cyst is entered it can be outlined by injecting a small quantity of contrast medium. This will show the size of the cyst and the contrast can be used to confirm that most or all of the fluid has been aspirated.

Ultrasound

The kidneys are well shown by ultrasound which has the valuable property of distinguishing between renal solid masses and renal cysts (Figs 10.10, 10.11 and 10.12). Cysts can also be localised by ultrasound for percutaneous puncture. Hydronephrosis is also well demonstrated by ultrasound as are polycystic kidneys. In the field of renal transplantation ultrasound is valuable in showing perirenal fluid and lymph collections (lymphoceles) and confirming swelling of the kidneys associated with rejection.

The distended *bladder* is well shown by abdominal ultrasound and tumours including infiltration of the wall can be assessed. The *prostate* can also be demonstrated, but is best shown by endoscopic transrectal ultrasound. This is now widely used for ultrasound guided biopsy of prostatic lesions.

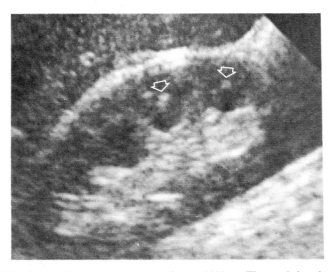

Fig. 10.10 Longitudinal ultrasound scan of normal kidney. The renal sinus is echogenic. The pyramids are relatively hypoechoic compared with the remainder of the parenchyma. The dense echoes (arrows) at the bases of the pyramids are due to the arcuate arteries.

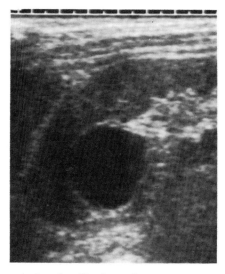

Fig. 10.11 Parasagittal section. Simple renal cyst.

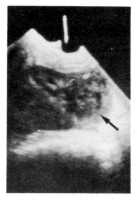

Fig. 10.12 Renal cell carcinoma of right kidney. Prone longitudinal scan. The lower pole of the kidney is bulbous. The central echo pattern is destroyed and the mass (arrow) contains multiple echoes arising from within the tumour. The outline of the mass is poorly defined.

Isotope scanning

$^{99}Tc^m$ DMSA (dimercaptosuccinic acid) is widely used for renal imaging. This compound is fixed in the tubules with a low extraction rate and good images may be obtained 1 to 2 hours after injection.

Lesions such as tumours show as filling defects as do benign lesions such as cysts (Fig. 10.13). In chronic pyelonephritis uptake is often reduced and uneven as it is in other conditions with poor renal function, such as obstructive uropathy and tuberculosis.

Renography. This method of scanning is widely used in renal disease. It differs from normal scanning in that a graph is obtained of the renal output of the isotope. The radioisotope used is usually ^{131}I hippuran or ^{123}I hippuran. This is removed almost entirely from the kidney in one passage and is not reabsorbed. Scanning must therefore take place immediately after a small intravenous injection of the radioactive isotope. A scintillator counter is centred evenly over each kidney touching the skin. The normal renogram graph usually shows (Fig. 10.14).

1. A sharp rise of activity within 30 seconds of the injection (A–B)
2. A slower rise during the next 3 to 5 minutes (B–C)
3. Falling off in the next 15 minutes (C–D)

This is the normal pattern but it will be changed in various ways depending on the type of disease from which the kidney is suffering. Comparison of the function of the two kidneys is also possible by comparing the results on the two sides.

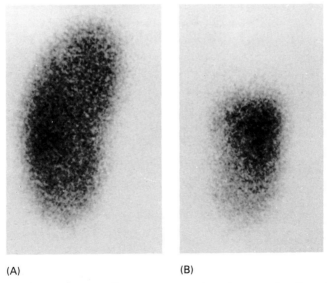

(A)   (B)

Fig. 10.13   Right renal cyst. [99]Tc^m DMSA scan. Posterior projection. Normal left image. There is a non-specific deficit in the upper half of the right kidney due to a cyst.

CT

Tumours, cysts and various other lesions of the kidneys are all well shown. CT is particularly valuable in the patient with a non-functioning kidney in demonstrating the cause. It may even prove whether a kidney is present or not when this remains doubtful by other techniques. It will readily differentiate between renal tumours and cysts (Fig. 10.15) and is invaluable for the staging of renal tumours (Fig. 10.16).

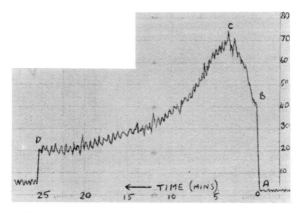

Fig. 10.14 ¹³¹I hippuran renogram. Normal. For explanation see text.

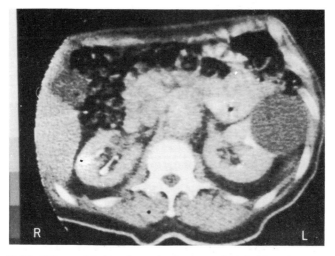

Fig. 10.15 CT scan showing a large simple cyst on the left side and a small simple cyst on the right side.

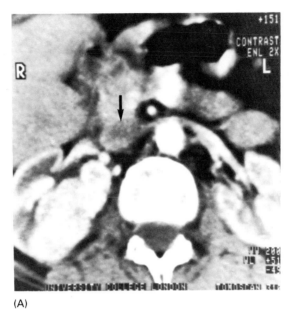

(A)

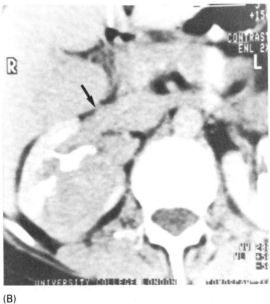

(B)

Fig. 10.16   A. Vascular carcinoma of right kidney showing marked but transient, enhancement. Note tumour thrombus in IVC (arrow). B. Later scan shows tumour enhancing less than renal tissue and a dilated occluded right renal vein (arrow).

The adrenals

Imaging of the adrenals is mainly undertaken for the demonstration of suspected mass lesions. These are listed in Table 10.1. They may be large or small and both may be endocrine functioning or non-functioning. The larger masses are more likely to be malignant tumours.

Endocrine functioning tumours of the adrenal can present with several different clinical syndromes. *Cushing's syndrome, Conn's syndrome* and the *adreno-genital syndrome* may all be seen with adenomas and less commonly with carcinomas.

Table 10.1 Adrenal mass lesions

A. Neoplasms	B. Other mass lesions

1. Cortical
    Adenoma carcinoma
	1. Granuloma
	    Tuberculoma
	    Histoplasmosis

2. Medullary
    Neuroblastoma
    Ganglioneuroma
    Phaeochromocytoma
	2. Cysts
	3. Haematomas

3. Stromal
    Lipoma
    Myolipoma
	4. Amyloid
	5. Bilateral hyperplasia

4. Metastases	

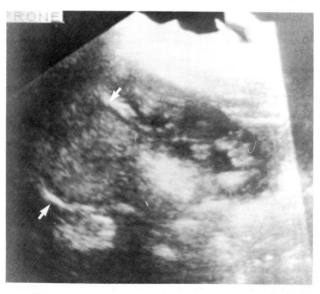

Fig. 10.17 Ultrasound scan shows large rounded tumour (arrows) above upper pole of right kidney.

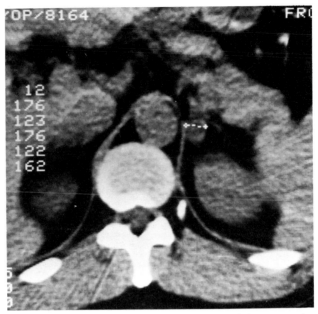

Fig. 10.18 Left-sided Conn's tumour seen as small rounded mass anterior to the upper pole of the left kidney. The superimposed electronic rule shows it measures 1.2 cm in diameter.

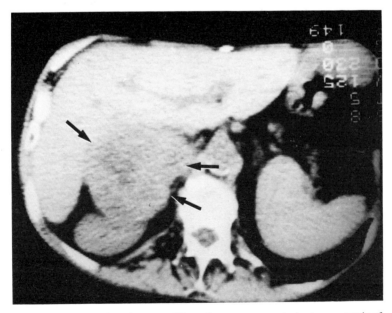

Fig. 10.19 Large adrenal tumour. Phaeochromocytoma anterior to upper pole of right kidney.

Cushing's syndrome may also be associated with bilateral hyperplasia as may the adreno-genital syndrome.

Phaeochromocytoma can give rise to adrenalism and noradrenalism.

Addison's disease can be due to bilateral granulomas but is now most commonly seen as the result of auto-immune disease.

Non-functioning tumours will only present clinically when large enough to produce a clinically palpable mass or when shown accidentally at imaging for other purposes. Large non-functioning tumours are more likely to be malignant – carcinoma in adults and neuroblastoma in children.

Imaging. Large tumours may be shown by *simple X-ray* or at IVP as masses displacing the kidney downwards. They are also readily seen at *ultrasound* examination (Fig. 10.17).

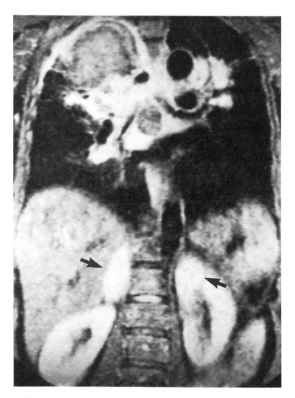

Fig. 10.20 Coronal MRI scan (T_2-weighted) shows bilateral adrenal metastases (arrows) as high-signal masses. Primary lung carcinoma with collapse of right upper lobe is also well shown. (Courtesy of Dr Gordon Thomson and Bristol MRI Centre.)

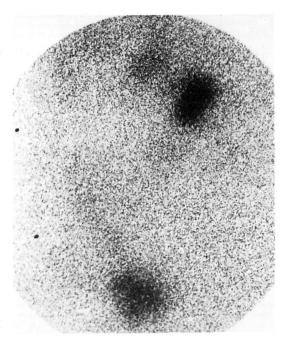

Fig. 10.21 ^{131}I-meta-iodo-benzyl-guanidine (MIBG) scan. Phaeochromocytoma. In the upper abdomen there are two foci of activity, the lateral one being more intense. They correspond to the site of a known malignant tumour of the left adrenal with adjacent lymph node involvement. Note there is bladder activity due to excretion of free iodine.

Small tumours, such as the small adenomas usually responsible for Conn's syndrome, are best identified by CT as are most medium sized masses (Figs 10.18 and 10.19). MRI can also show such masses well (Fig. 10.20).

Phaeochromocytomas may present special problems as some 10% are ectopic in position and can arise in sympathetic tissue remote from the adrenal. In such cases *venous sampling* for raised catecholamine values in different areas may help localisation and *isotope scanning* may prove helpful in localising the tumour. It is also valuable for the demonstration of metastases in the small proportion of phaeochromocytomas which are multiple or malignant. Metaiodobenzylguanidine (MIBG) labelled with radioactive ^{131}I or ^{123}I is the isotope used (Fig. 10.21). The same drug can be used in isotope scanning of neuroblastomas.

11. Obstetrics and gynaecology

OBSTETRICS

Ultrasound found its first major clinical usage in obstetrics and has made its greatest contribution in this field. It is now the vital technique for the monitoring of normal and abnormal pregnancy.

Early pregnancy (first trimester)

The normal non pregnant uterus at transabdominal scanning is shown as an egg-shaped structure, larger at the fundus, and lying directly behind the distended bladder (Fig. 11.1). All pelvic ultrasound examinations should be conducted with the bladder well distended, as this displaces gas-containing bowel and allows uninterrupted access of the ultrasound beam to the uterus lying behind the bladder.

In early pregnancy the uterus enlarges and a gestation sac can be identified as early as 5–6 weeks after the first day of the last menstrual period. Transvaginal scanning can identity the sac as early as 4 weeks. It appears as a cystic area with a rim of high intensity echoes. By 10 weeks the sac has enlarged to occupy most of the uterine cavity (Figs 11.2 and 11.3). The developing embryo or 'fetal node' can be identified from the 6th or 7th week and the fetal head at 14 weeks. Multiple pregnancy can also be identified at an early stage by the presence of two or more gestation sacs (Fig. 11.4).

The *fetal heart beat* can be identified soon after the fetal node is seen and must always be looked for as evidence of a live fetus.

The *crown rump length* of the fetal node can be measured accurately by electronic calipers between the 7th and 14th weeks of pregnancy and assessed against the normal standards. In a normal pregnancy the measurement can predict maturity with considerable

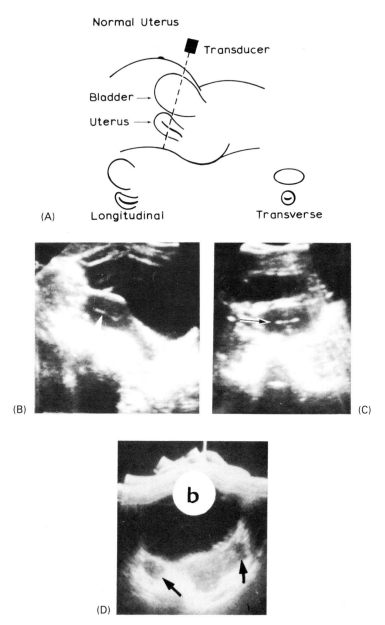

Fig. 11.1 (A) Diagram indicating the position of the ultrasound transducer, the patient's abdominal wall, bladder and uterus. (B) Longitudinal scan showing the structures indicated in Figure 11.1A. The arrow indicates the uterine cavity. (C) Uterine cavity (arrowed) shown on transverse scan. (D) Transverse scan showing the ovaries (arrowed), on each side of the uterus, behind the filled bladder (**b**).

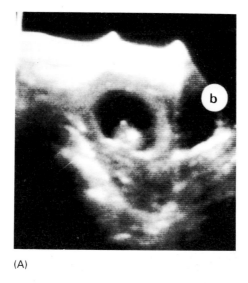

(A)

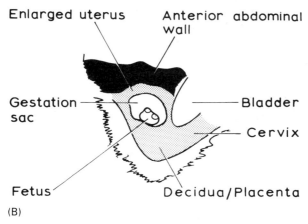

(B)

Fig. 11.2 Early pregnancy. (A) Longitudinal scan. 9 weeks menstrual age. The gestation sac is large at this stage and the fetus (fetal node) is shown as an oval collection of echoes within it. **b** = bladder. (B) Diagram of (A).

accuracy. *Gestation sac volume* can also be measured by ultrasound but is less accurate in assessing maturity.

Abnormalities of early pregnancy

These include:

1. Missed abortion

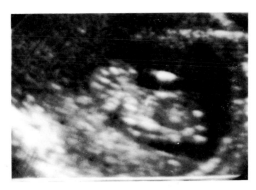

Fig. 11.3 Pregnancy at 10 weeks and 3 days. The crown rump length can easily be measured by electronic calipers.

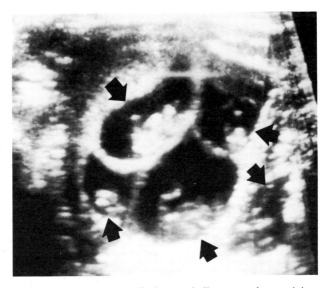

Fig. 11.4 Quintuplet pregnancy. Each arrow indicates a node-containing gestation sac.

2. Anembryonic pregnancy (blighted ovum)
3. Live abortion
4. Hydatidiform mole
5. Ectopic pregnancy.

Missed abortion accounts for nearly half the cases of early pregnancy failure. At ultrasound the fetal heart beat cannot be detected even with real-time scanning. It is important to realise that even with a dead fetus it is still possible to have a positive pregnancy test as the trophoblast can continue to function.

Anembryonic pregnancy is almost as common as missed abortion. The diagnosis is made in those pregnancies in which the gestation sac cannot be shown to contain a fetus either at ultrasound (Fig. 11.5) or in the aborted products of gestation. Apart from this absence of a fetal node and fetal heart beat the gestation sac is 'small for dates' at ultrasound.

Live abortion is defined as *early* (before 12th week) or *late* (after 12th week). The early group may show a low gestation sac volume at ultrasound but appearances may be normal even a few days before abortion.

Hydatidiform mole is rare in Europe (about 1 in 2000 pregnancies). At ultrasound the uterus is large for dates. No fetal parts or fetal heart beat can be detected, and the uterus is full of multiple fine echoes (Fig. 11.6). The patients have high gonadotrophic levels in the urine.

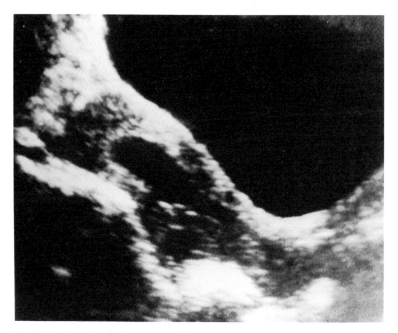

Fig. 11.5 Anembryonic pregnancy. The uterus and sac lie behind the distended bladder. They are small for dates and no fetal node is identified.

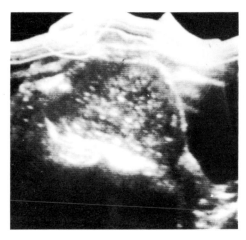

Fig. 11.6 Hydatidiform mole, 17th week of amenorrhoea. The uterus is enlarged and there are multiple echoes within it of high and low echogenicity. No fetal parts visible and no fetal pulsations detectable.

Ectopic pregnancy. This may be *unruptured* in which case the gestation sac is identified in an extra-uterine location and a fetal node and fetal heart beat are identified within it, or it may be *ruptured* in which case the extra-uterine sac is associated with a complex haematoma mass. In both cases the uterus is enlarged and contains a mottled pattern but no gestation sac. Diagnosis of the adnexal mass can be difficult and in some cases may require laparoscopy.

Mid and late pregnancy (second and third trimesters)

18 to 20 weeks is a good time to perform routine examination of pregnancy by ultrasound. This should document:

1. Fetal number
2. Fetal life (heart beat)
3. Fetal position
4. Gestational age (see below)
5. Abnormalities of the fetus (see below)
6. Placental location
7. Amniotic fluid – normal, polyhydramnios or oligohydramnios.

Fetal age

Various parameters can be used for assessing fetal age. The measurements are then compared with standard charts based on large series. The measurements used are:

1. Biparietal diameter of the skull (BPD)
2. Femoral length (FL)
3. Head circumference (HC)
4. Abdominal circumference (AC).

Crown–rump length is also used in the early stages of pregnancy (up to 9 or 10 weeks) and before the other parameters are readily usable.

The measurements listed are accurate ± 1 to 2 weeks in the first and second trimester but only ± 2 to 3 weeks nearer term.

The BPD is perhaps most widely used and is measured on a transverse axial image of the skull at its widest diameter (Fig. 11.7).

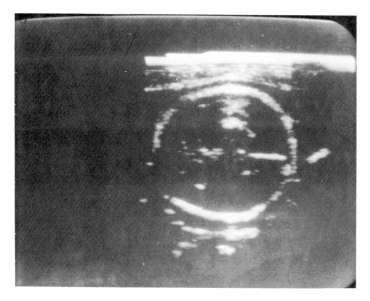

Fig. 11.7 Fetal head showing correct position for measuring biparietal diameter. The midline falx echo is clearly seen.

Genetic screening

Amniocentesis, chorionic villous sampling and fetal blood sampling are invasive procedures which are being increasingly used for genetic screening. They all require ultrasound control for success, and carry a risk of fetal loss or damage.

Maternal serum fetoprotein (MSAFP) screening is a useful non-invasive test which can be helpful in selecting patients for the more invasive procedures at 15 to 20 weeks.

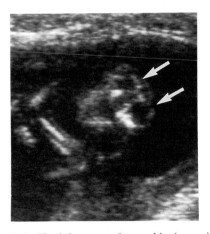

Fig. 11.8   Anencephaly. Head shows prominent orbits (arrows) but no cerebral tissues or vault above.

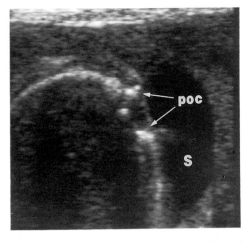

Fig. 11.9   Meningocoele: transverse image. S = sac containing only fluid, poc = splaying of the posterior ossification centres.

Fetal abnormalities

Many congenital abnormalities of the fetus can now be recognised in utero by ultrasound screening. In many cases these can be recognised sufficiently early for therapeutic termination to be a realistic possibility where this is considered desirable.

Neural tube defects. These include the fatal condition of *anencephaly* (Fig. 11.8) and the various forms of *spina bifida* ranging from severe lumbar myelomeningocele to potentially correctable meningocele (Fig. 11.9). Encephalocele, hydrocephalus and various congenital anomalies of the brain are all identifiable.

Thorax. Heart. A four chamber view of the fetal heart can be obtained from about 18 weeks onwards (Fig. 11.10). Not only can the cardiac chambers and great vessels be measured but dysrhythmias and valvular lesions can be diagnosed and the latter quantified using colour Doppler. Thus many forms of congenital heart disease and other cardiac anomalies can now be diagnosed in utero.

Congenital diaphragmatic hernia (CDH) is a rare but serious condition which can also be recognised in utero as can other rare congenital lung anomalies.

Abdomen. Abdominal wall defects leading to omphalocele or gastroschisis have been diagnosed at fetal ultrasound as have duodenal atresia, ascites and other anomalies. Lesions of the GU system recognised include the fatal bilateral renal agenesis (Potter's syndrome or reno-facial dysplasia), infantile renal polycystic dis-

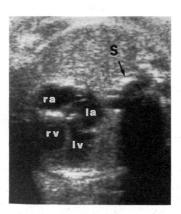

Fig. 11.10 Fetal heart: subcostal four-chamber image. S = spine, ra = right atrium, la = left atrium, rv = right ventricle with moderator band, lv = left ventricle.

ease and multicystic dysplastic kidneys. Fetal hydronephrosis, unilateral and bilateral, is also diagnosable.

Hydrops fetalis due to isoimmunisation from feto-maternal blood group incompatibility is now rare since it can be treated by Rh-immune globulin therapy. Most of the cases seen now are associated with non-immunological causes including a wide variety of fetal congenital and other abnormalities.

The sonographic features include:

1. Polyhydramnios (Fig. 11.11)
2. Increased placental thickness
3. Skin thickening
4. Ascites, pleural and pericardial effusion.

The placenta

The placenta is easily identified by ultrasound and its site is always noted at routine examination (Figs 11.12 and 11.13). Localisation is particularly important in:

1. Antepartum haemorrhage (placenta praevia, abruptio placentae)
2. Amniocentesis.

With amniocentesis ultrasound control enables the needle to be inserted into a pool of amniotic fluid without traversing the placenta or causing damage to the fetus.

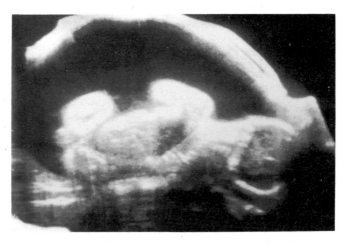

Fig. 11.11   Polyhydramnios; there is a gross excess of amniotic fluid.

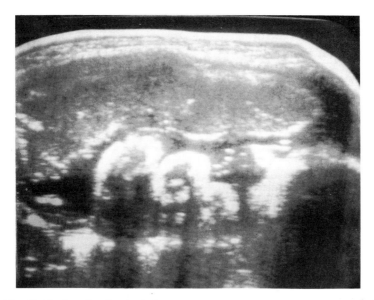

Fig. 11.12 Anterior placenta in late pregnancy.

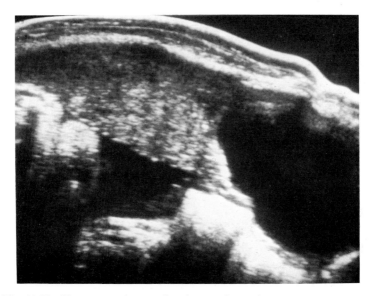

Fig. 11.13 Placenta praevia extending down to the cervix.

MRI

There is as yet no experimental or other evidence that MRI is harmful to the fetus but both the National Radiation Protection Board in the UK and the Food and Drugs Administration in the USA recommend that it should not be used in the first trimester.

GYNAECOLOGY

Ultrasound

Ultrasound of the female pelvis is now the primary imaging investigation in many gynaecological problems. These include the investigation of congenital anomalies, of pelvic masses and pelvic inflammatory disease, the monitoring of ovarian function and ovarian pathology, the assessment of uterine pathology, and the control of intra-uterine contraceptive devices (IUCD).

Most cases are examined by transabdominal scanning, but transvaginal scanning can provide better detail in selected cases as can transrectal scanning in elderly patients.

IUCDs. These are readily identified by ultrasound as a strong linear echo or a row of punctate echoes within the uterine cavity, sometimes with acoustic shadowing (Fig. 11.14). Where the IUCD is not shown a plain abdominal X-ray is required to exclude the rare complication of migration of the device into the abdominal cavity.

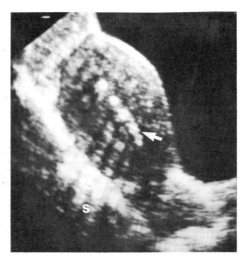

Fig. 11.14   IUCD (arrowed). Note acoustic shadowing (S).

Ovarian function. The normal ovaries can usually be identified as small ovoid structures lateral to the uterus and hypoechoic to the surrounding pelvic fat. They are largest in the post-pubertal female when they reach 3 × 2 cm or more in size, but atrophy in the post-menopausal female. Post puberty several tiny cysts may be seen in the peripheral zone of the ovary representing follicles.

During the menstrual cycle the development of a dominant follicle can be observed by ultrasound as it increases in size from less than 5 mm to as much as 20 mm in size. This takes place by day 14 when rupture occurs.

Enlarged ovaries with multiple cysts may be seen in the Stein–Leventhal syndrome (amenorrhoea, infertility, hirsutism and obesity). Multicystic ovaries may also be seen in anorexics and in athletes. They are also a feature of Pergonal stimulation in the treatment of infertility (Fig. 11.15).

Pelvic masses

Uterine fibroids are the commonest female tumour, occurring in 20% of females above the age of 30. They can be interstitial, submucosal or subserous in position and small or large in size. They can also undergo hyaline or cystic degeneration and they fre-

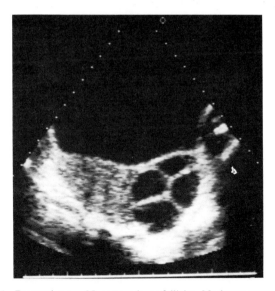

Fig. 11.15 Pergonal ovary. Numerous large follicles. Moderate overstimulation.

quently calcify. The sonographic features are equally diverse but they usually enlarge the uterus giving it a bulbous fundus and an irregular or lobulated contour. A focal uterine mass may show hypo- or hyper- echoic features. Calcification is markedly hyperechoic.

Uterine *carcinoma*, both endometrial and cervical, is best assessed by CT or MRI which are also valuable in staging. Primary diagnosis is rarely made by ultrasound but it can demonstrate the tumour mass and help in staging and in monitoring the results of treatment.

Hydatidiform mole and the rarer *choriocarcinoma* show characteristic features at sonography. The uterine cavity is occupied by a large echogenic mass which is homogeneous during the first trimester but develops small cystic cavities in the second trimester (Fig. 11.6).

Ovarian masses are often cystic. They include *cystadenoma, cystadenocarcinoma, dermoid, teratoma* and other rare tumours. In young females, benign tumours predominate by 5 to 1, but in post menopausal patients the incidence of malignancy rises to reach 2 to 1.

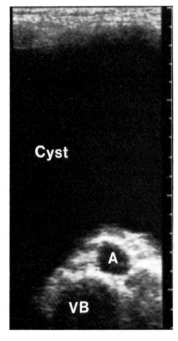

Fig. 11.16 The empty abdomen appearance caused by a huge cyst displacing the abdominal organs. Note aorta (A) and vertebral body (VB) are seen in horizontal section.

Cystadenomas at ultrasound usually appear as thin walled cysts. These can become very large giving rise in extreme cases to the sonographically 'empty abdomen' (Figs 11.16 and 11.17). The mucinous type are more likely to contain septations than the serous type. *Cystadenocarcinomas* are more likely to be complex cysts with solid components and ascites is often present (Fig. 11.18).

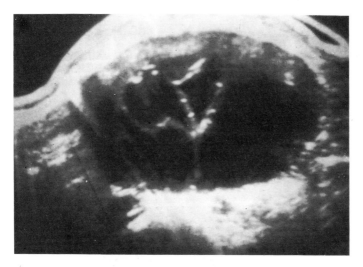

Fig. 11.17 Ovarian cyst with septa seen anteriorly.

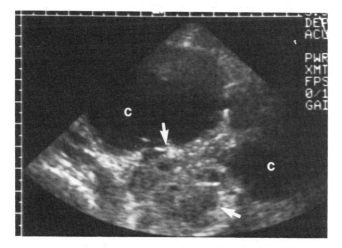

Fig. 11.18 Biloculated cystadenocarcinoma with a large solid component. c = cystic components, solid component arrowed.

CT and MRI

CT is now widely used in the further assessment of pelvic and abdominal tumours and is particularly valuable in the staging of malignant tumours (Fig. 11.19). MRI is probably more accurate than CT in the staging of uterine carcinomas, particularly cervical carcinoma (Fig. 11.20) but ovarian carcinoma is better staged by CT.

Simple X-ray

Simple X-rays of the pelvis can be helpful in the diagnosis and differential diagnosis of some pelvic masses in the female. *Fibroids*

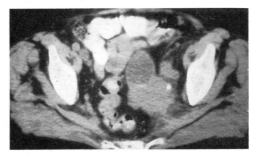

Fig. 11.19 Cystadenocarcinoma of the left ovary with a solid component extending to the pelvic side wall. Deep extension and distant nodal metastatic spread are better seen by CT than by ultrasonography.

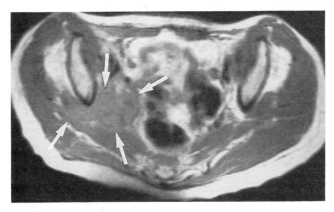

Fig. 11.20 Tumour infiltration (arrows) of the right pelvic side-wall, on a transverse T_1-weighted spin-echo (SE 70/40) image, in a patient with carcinoma of the cervix treated by hysterectomy 6 months previously.

often calcify and the calcification has a characteristic mottled irregular appearance on X-ray which is diagnostic (Fig. 11.21).

Ovarian dermoids may show calcification in their wall or they

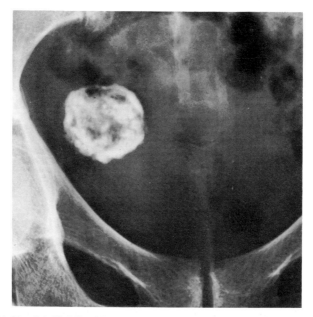

Fig. 11.21 Calcified fibroid.

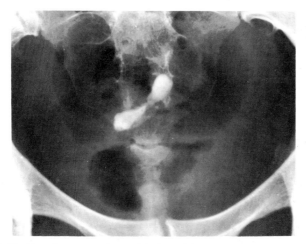

Fig. 11.22 Dental structures in a pelvic dermoid.

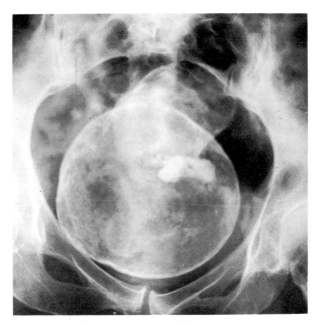

Fig. 11.23 Large calcified dermoid in the pelvis.

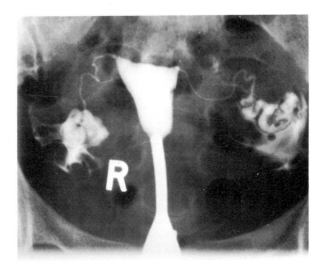

Fig. 11.24 Normal salpingogram, both Fallopian tubes fill and contrast is seen in the peritoneum. The ulterine cavity in also outlined.

may show dental structures which can be readily recognised by radiology (Figs 11.22 and 11.23). Occasionally, owing to their high fat content, a relative translucency within the tumour may be recognised. *Tuberculous pyosalpinx* may show characteristic calcareous debris outlining the lesion.

Apart from simple X-rays the only other X-ray technique still widely used for the investigation of gynaecological problems is *salpingography.*

Hysterosalpingography

Hysterosalpingography is most widely used in the investigation of sterility. The investigation is obviously contraindicated in the presence of pregnancy, severe haemorrhage or active infection.

With water soluble contrast media peritoneal spill from the tubes can be observed immediately by screening the salpingogram during

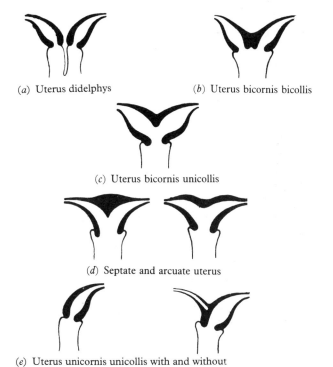

(*a*) Uterus didelphys (*b*) Uterus bicornis bicollis

(*c*) Uterus bicornis unicollis

(*d*) Septate and arcuate uterus

(*e*) Uterus unicornis unicollis with and without rudimentary opposite horns

Fig. 11.25 Diagrammatic representation of important congenital abnormalities of the uterus.

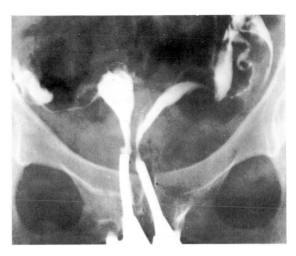

Fig. 11.26   Uterus bicornis bicollis.

injection. Salpingography is performed in the X-ray department and is best done by the radiologist and gynaecologist in cooperation. The radiologist observes the injection on an image intensifier and takes any appropriate pictures necessary.

The normal hysterosalpingogram (Fig. 11.24) shows the uterus as an inverted triangular shadow and the tubes as fine sinuous lines extending out from the cornual angles.

In cases of sterility normal appearances may be shown with a free spill into the peritoneum and a local mechanical cause may thus be excluded. In these normal cases the prognosis is fair and in one series about a third of the patients subsequently became pregnant. It has even been postulated that salpingography had a therapeutic effect in some of these patients by clearing adhesions. On the other hand the salpingogram may show a definite cause for sterility such as blockage of both tubes or the presence of bilateral hydrosalpinx. Congenital anomalies of the uterus such as bicornuate or infantile uterus may be seen, or grosser anomalies such as uterus didelphys may be diagnosed (Figs 11.25 and 11.26).

12. Neuroradiology

Imaging of the skull, spine and central nervous system utilises techniques which permit a remarkable accuracy in pathological and anatomical diagnosis. These include:

1. Simple X-ray and tomography
2. Angiography
   a. Carotid arteriography
   b. Vertebral arteriography
   c. Arch aortography
   d. Spinal angiography
   e. Digital vascular imaging (DVI)
3. Myelography and radiculography
4. Isotope scanning
5. CT
6. MRI
7. Ultrasound.

The newer techniques have helped to change radically the accuracy of diagnosis, the prognosis and the treatment in many neurological conditions. This is particularly so in the field of tumours and vascular lesions where the introduction of CT in 1972 initiated a new era in radiological diagnosis.

Choice of investigation

Nearly all patients with suspected intracranial lesions are now examined first by CT or MRI with or without a preliminary simple skull X-ray. In many cases this will establish the diagnosis or, if tumour is suspected, will exclude the possibility of tumour. *Angiography* has a valuable role to play, particularly in the elucidation of vascular lesions. It may also be occasionally required to further elucidate the pathology and blood supply of a tumour shown at

CT or MRI. Isotope scanning once widely practised is now rarely performed where CT is also available.

In neonates and small infants it is possible to examine the brain and ventricles by *ultrasound* using the 'window' provided by the open fontanelle and many lesions can thus be diagnosed (Fig. 12.1). Unfortunately the technique cannot be used in the same way for adults and older children because of the skull barrier. However, Doppler ultrasound is used in adults for screening carotid bifurcations in suspected atheromatous stenosis.

MRI has proved superior to CT in the demonstration of demyelinating diseases such as MS, and is also superior in the delineation of many posterior fossa lesions. As techniques improve it is likely to further supplant CT.

Plain radiography

Plain radiography of the skull may show evidence of a cerebral tumour either in a general manner or, less commonly, in a manner permitting accurate localisation. The general evidence of cerebral tumour consists of changes in the skull induced by the chronic raised intracranial pressure. In children the most important of these is suture diastasis (Fig. 12.2); in the adult it is thinning or erosion of the dorsum sellae (Fig. 12.3). So-called 'increased

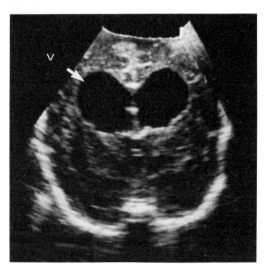

Fig. 12.1   Ultrasound coronal section in an infant showing hydrocephalus. V = dilated lateral ventricle.

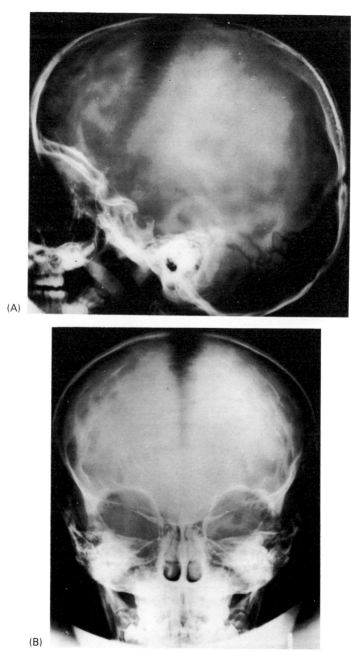

(A)

(B)

Fig. 12.2 Lateral and PA skull films of child with raised intracranial pressure and marked suture diastasis involving the coronal and sagittal sutures.

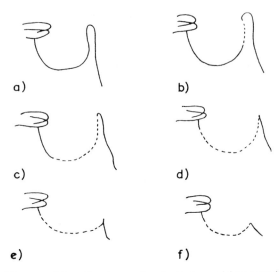

a)   b)

c)   d)

e)   f)

Fig. 12.3 Diagram of the sellar changes in raised intracranial pressure in the adult. (*a*) to (*f*) show progressive changes from slight in (*b*) to gross in (*f*).

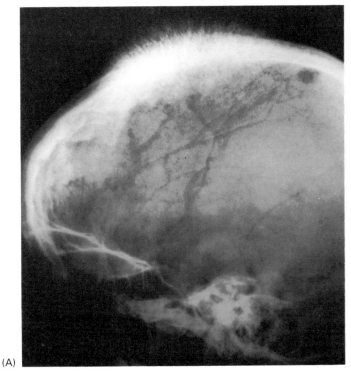

(A)

Fig. 12.4(A)

convolutional markings' or 'copper beating' of the skull vault is now generally considered to be of little diagnostic importance.

Localising evidence of the presence of a cerebral tumour may manifest as local erosion of the skull vault; thus a *pituitary adenoma* may expand and 'balloon' the sella, and an *acoustic neurinoma* may expand and erode an internal auditory meatus. Both these changes can be demonstrated by plain X-rays as can erosions in the skull vault by metastases. Lateral displacement of the calcified pineal gland is another important radiological sign often observed in adults with tumours in a cerebral hemisphere. Local bony thickening or hyperostosis is not infrequently seen with meningiomas, particularly in their common parasagittal or sphenoidal ridge localisation (Fig. 12.4).

Intracranial *calcification* is seen with a small proportion of intracranial tumours. Cerebral *gliomas* form about half the tumours seen

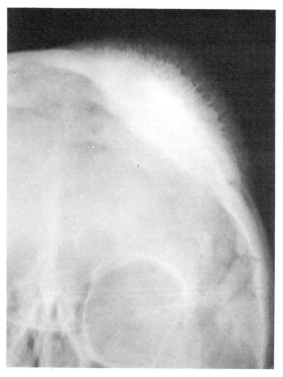

(B)

Fig. 12.4 Meningioma growing through the skull vault. Note the sun-ray spiculation and the enlarged vascular channels of the skull vault. (A) Lateral view. (B) PA view.

in clinical practice; about 7% of these will show calcification in the tumour enabling a localisation to be made on plain X-ray. *Meningiomas* calcify in some 10% of cases, whilst *craniopharyngiomas*, presenting in children, show calcification in over 70% of cases (Fig. 12.5). Tumour calcification has to be distinguished from the calcification seen in various other conditions. The calcification in many of these is pathognomonic. For instance, the sinuous tramline occipital calcification seen in the *Sturge–Weber syndrome* or the ring calcification seen in a small proportion of *cerebral aneurysms*.

Although plain X-rays are helpful in some cases and may prove diagnostic in a few, further specialised investigation is necessary with most suspected tumours for accurate localisation and for further assistance towards diagnosis before a neurosurgeon performs a craniotomy. Generally speaking, the primary method of

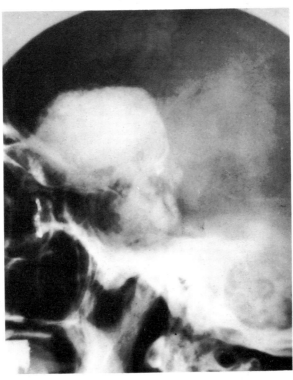

Fig. 12.5 Heavily calcified craniopharyngioma growing upwards and forwards from the sella.

investigation will be the least traumatic and invasive. This will be CT scanning or MRI if available.

Cerebral angiography

The widespread use of angiography revolutionised the diagnosis and treatment of vascular lesions affecting the cerebral circulation. *Cerebral aneurysms,* whether presenting in their most common manner as subarachnoid haemorrhage or in other ways, are now routinely investigated by arteriography (Fig. 12.6).

The possibility of localising and defining the source of a *subarachnoid haemorrhage* stimulated attempts to improve the grave mortality and morbidity of this distressing condition by surgical means. The treatment of subarachnoid haemorrhage remains a controversial problem, but present views are in favour of surgical methods of treatment and most expert opinion now favours early radiological investigation by arteriography. Only thus can the source of a subarachnoid haemorrhage be clearly demonstrated and curative surgical treatment planned.

Cerebral *angiomas* or vascular malformations, formerly thought to be rare conditions, were shown by arteriography to be extremely

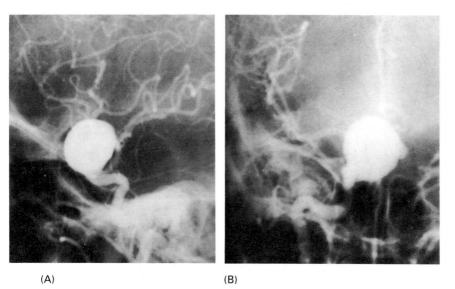

(A) (B)

Fig. 12.6 Large aneurysm which presented as a suprasellar mass. (A) Lateral view. (B) AP view.

common. These lesions are amenable in many cases to surgical treatment and can be totally removed by the neurosurgeon.

Thrombosis or embolic occlusion of major intracranial vessels can also be readily shown by arteriography. The syndrome of thrombosis of the internal carotid artery is now well recognised and the lesion is clearly demonstrated by arteriography (Fig. 12.7). Thrombosis usually occurs near the origin of the internal carotid artery which is a common site for atheromatous stenosis of the vessel. Such stenosis by an atheromatous plaque is also well shown by angiography, and may prove the explanation for remittent hemiplegia, or *transient ischaemic attacks* (TIAs). Obstruction to the cerebral blood flow produced by internal carotid stenosis is now treated surgically with a high degree of success.

It has been shown that similar stenotic lesions may occur at the origin of the vertebral artery and give rise to *vertebro-basilar insufficiency*. These lesions can also be shown radiologically using percutaneous catheter techniques and *arch aortography* or *DSA*.

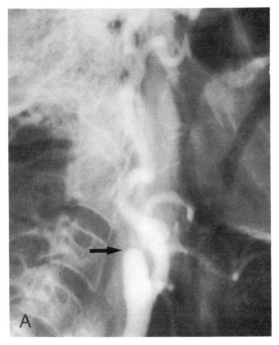

Fig. 12.7(A)

Other vascular lesions such as *subdural haematoma* and *intracerebral haematoma* can also be demonstrated by angiography but are less invasively shown by CT or MRI.

DVI (DSA)

Digital vascular imaging (DVI) is now quite widely used for the assessment of suspected carotid stenosis or thrombosis. This technique uses computers to subtract bone and other tissues from the contrast enhanced blood vessels. The contrast can be injected intravenously and the patient examined on an outpatient basis (Fig. 12.8).

CT and MRI

The clinical usage of both these revolutionary techniques was pioneered in neuroradiology. Both began in Britain, CT in 1972

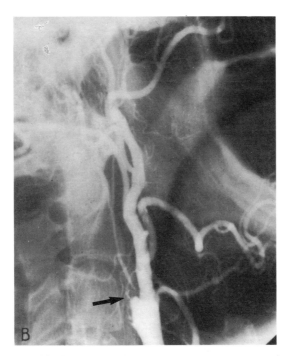

Fig. 12.7 (A and B) Thrombosis of the internal carotid artery in the neck. The external carotid is patent. Two different cases.

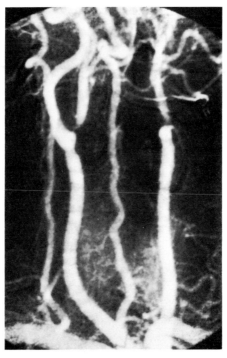

Fig. 12.8   Neck vessels shown by intravenous DVI. There are bilateral stenoses at the internal carotid origins.

and MRI in 1981. The student should be familiar with the appearances of the brain in axial CT sections (Fig. 12.9), and should be able to identify the normal structures illustrated. MRI can already improve on the resolution achieved by CT and has the advantage of easily producing sagittal and coronal sections. However it is much more expensive and is less widely available.

Congenital lesions

Large heads in infants and children are usually due to hydrocephalus, though there are other rare causes such as congenital large brains (macrocephaly), leukodystrophy or storage diseases.

Hydrocephalus. This may be *communicating* or *non-communicating* depending on the obstruction being within the brain or in the subarachnoid space. The level of obstruction can be diagnosed at CT or MRI. In childhood most of the non-communicating cases are due to aqueduct stenosis, the Dandy Walker syndrome or to

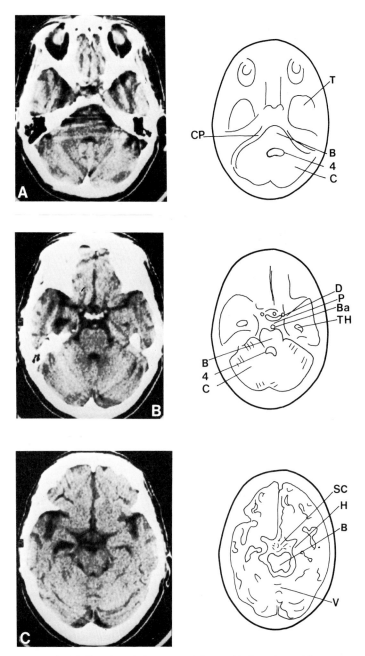

Fig. 12.9 Serial slices from below upwards in an elderly patient with some degree of atrophy with diagrams to illustrate normal anatomy. (Key on p. 221.)

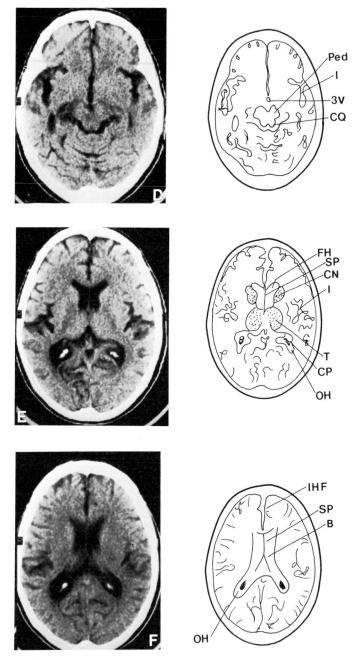

Fig. 12.9 (*contd*) Key on page 221.

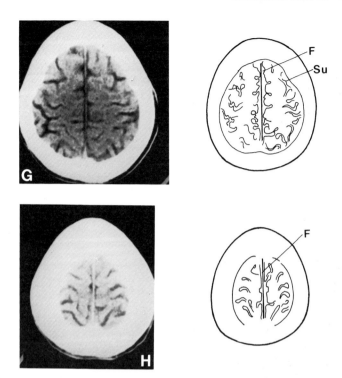

Fig. 12.9 (*contd*)   Serial slices from below upwards in an elderly patient with some degree of atrophy with diagrams to illustrate normal anatomy. **A** T–temporal lobe, CP–cerebellopontine angle, B–brainstem, 4–4th ventricle, C–cerebellum. **B** D–dorsum sellae, P–pontine cistern, Ba–basilar artery, TH–temporal horn. **C** SC–suprasellar cistern, H–hippocampus, B–brainstem, V–vermis. **D** Ped–peduncle, I–insula, 3V–3rd ventricle, CQ–corpora quadrigemina. **E** FH–frontal horn, SP–septum pellucidum, CN–caudate nucleus, T–thalamus, CP–choroid plexus, OH–occipital horn. **F** IHF–interhemispheric fissure, B–body of lateral ventricle. **G** Su–sulci, F–falx.

arachnoid cysts. About one-third of the cases in children may be communicating and these are secondary to subarachnoid haemorrhage or meningitis, leading to obstruction of the c.s.f. flow in the subarachnoid space and basal cisterns.

Hydrocephalus may also be seen in spina bifida and spinal dysraphism when it is associated with a Chiari type 2 malformation of the brain stem (caudal displacement of the pons, medulla, and fourth ventricle).

Aqueduct stenosis is a congenital condition obstructing the flow of c.s.f. and leading to dilatation of the third and lateral ventricles with enlargement of the head. It usually presents in infancy or childhood but occasionally is not recognised or manifest until adult life. The *Dandy Walker* syndrome is also a congenital condition in which there is obstruction to the outflow of c.s.f. from the 4th ventricle, associated with varying degrees of cystic dilatation of the 4th ventricle and dilatation of the ventricles above.

Intracranial tumours

Tumours within the skull may be either *intracerebral* or *extracerebral*. This distinction is important with respect to treatment and prognosis, since most intracranial tumours are malignant and most extracranial ones are benign. In a pathological series *gliomas* formed 31% of the intracranial tumours and *metastases* 20% (see Table 12.1).

Table 12.1 Distribution of tumours in a pathological series (5199 cases – after Zimmerman, 1971)

	%		%
Glioma	31.0	Blood vessel tumours	6.0
Meningioma	15.0	Congenital tumours	2.0
Pit. adenoma	5.0	Metastatic	21.0
Acoustic	1.5	Granuloma	6.0
		Miscellaneous	12.5

At CT scanning most gliomas show areas of mixed attenuation within the brain displacing and deforming the ventricles. After intravenous contrast injection the tumour may show patchy en-

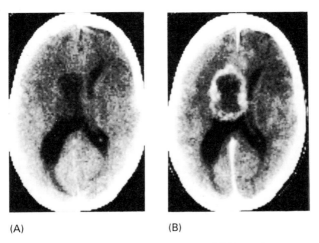

(A)   (B)

Fig. 12.10 Cystic glioma. (A) Before enhancement. (B) Postenhancement (L36 W80).

hancement of varying degrees or it may show irregular ring enhancement. Figures 12.10–12.13 show gliomas of different types and their appearances at CT scanning.

Metastases vary greatly in their CT appearances. They may show reduced or increased attenuation and the majority show obvious enhancement after intravenous contrast medium, often as a small ring shadow. There may be considerable surrounding oedema shown as a low density area. This diagnosis is made more certain

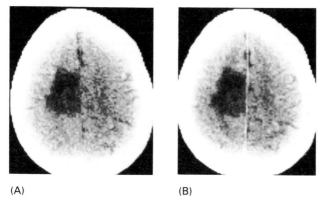

(A) (B)

Fig. 12.11 Low grade glioma. (A) Low attenuation parasagittal area with no mass effect in axial cut. (B) No enhancement after contrast.

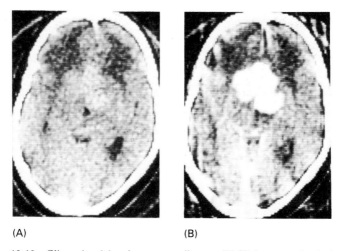

(A) (B)

Fig. 12.12 Glioma involving the corpus callosum. (A) High attenuation lesion. (B) Enhancing strongly with contrast. Oedema of frontal lobes (L30 W80).

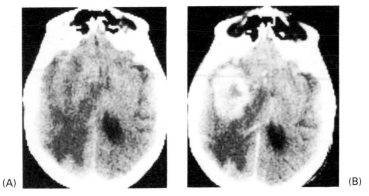

Fig. 12.13 Malignant glioma. (A) Mixed attenuation lesion with much oedema posteriorly in the white matter. (B) Marked enhancement of tumour after contrast (L30 W100).

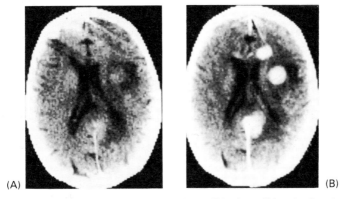

Fig. 12.14 Metastases. Three separate lesions, all isodense (A) and enhancing strongly with contrast (B). Oedema around the larger secondaries shown as low density areas. (L40 W60).

by the demonstration of multiple lesions widely scattered in the brain (see Fig.12.14).

Extracerebral tumours

These include meningiomas, acoustic tumours, dermoids, epidermoids, pituitary tumours and craniopharyngiomas.

Meningiomas tend to arise in characteristic sites and this fact coupled with a fairly typical CT appearance facilitates correct diagnosis. Favourite sites are the parasagittal region or over the cerebral convexity. The sphenoid ridge, the tuberculum sellae, and the cribriform plate are also common sites. Meningiomas appear as rounded lesions usually of increased density as compared with normal brain and sometimes containing calcifications. Most meningiomas enhance strongly after intravenous contrast injection (see Fig. 12.15).

Acoustic tumours also show typical appearances, usually appearing of low density but enhancing after contrast (Fig. 12.16A). Very small tumours are more difficult to demonstrate but can be outlined following the injection by lumbar puncture of a few ml of air (air meatography) (Fig. 12.16B) or water soluble contrast (cisternography). They can also be shown non-invasively by MRI (Fig. 12.24).

Vascular lesions

CT has revolutionised the non-invasive diagnosis of 'strokes' and is the most worthwhile form of primary investigation in any patient who has suffered or is suspected of suffering from a cerebrovascular accident. *Intracranial haemorrhage* or haematoma is shown as a high density lesion (Fig. 12.17) due to the clot. As the clot absorbs, the lesion becomes isodense and later of low attenuation. This residual low density represents the area of damaged brain. *Extracerebral haematoma*, both *extradural* and *subdural*, are well demonstrated, particularly in the acute phase, as high density peripheral lesions. Subdural haematoma may go through an isodense phase as the blood clot is absorbed and later becomes hypodense. Chronic subdural haematomas show a very characteristic appearance of a low density peripheral lesion in the skull (Fig. 12.18).

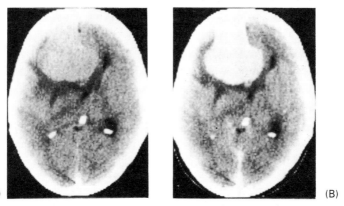

(A)   (B)

Fig. 12.15 (A) Frontal meningioma. High density tumour with some surrounding oedema. (B) Marked enhancement of tumour after contrast (L44 W80).

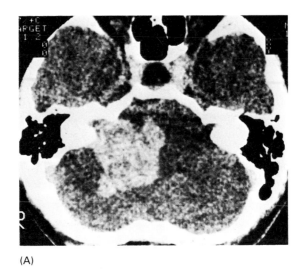

(A)

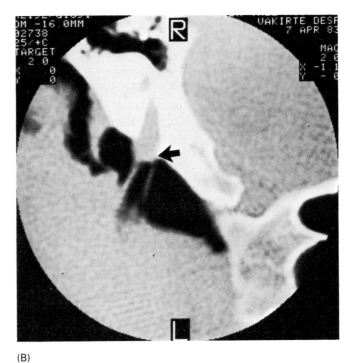

(B)

Fig. 12.16   (A) Large acoustic tumour postenhancement. (B) CT air meatogram shows small acoustic tumour just protruding from the meatus (←). The 7th and 8th nerves are also outlined by air.

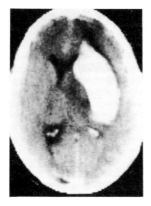

Fig. 12.17 Intracerebral haematoma. Massive capsular haemorrhage shown as white area (L36 W80).

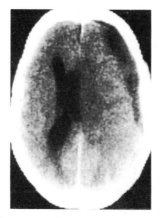

Fig. 12.18 Subdural haematoma three weeks after onset. The clot is largely absorbed and the subdural fluid is now of low density (L40 W80).

CT also provides an ideal non-invasive method of investigating patients with head injuries and comatose patients suspected of head injury. Apart from showing extradural and subdural haematomas, intracranial contusions with haemorrhage are also well shown as are the relationships of depressed fractures to underlying brain.

Subarachnoid haemorrhage is best investigated by CT in the first place. In a high proportion of cases the localisation of blood in the subarachnoid space or of secondary intracranial haematoma will establish where the ruptured aneurysm or angioma is sited. Large angiomas and aneurysms are also well shown by CT before they rupture, particularly after enhancement.

Cerebral thrombosis or embolus with infarction can be identified by CT. The affected area will show changes soon after infarction, usually of decreased attenuation, and often enhances with contrast. Later as the infarct becomes established the affected area shows as a low density lesion with no mass effect (Fig. 12.19).

Cerebral atrophy and other degenerative disorders are also well demonstrated by CT (Fig. 12.9), as are *inflammatory lesions* such as brain abscess or herpes encephalitis.

MRI

MRI can show most *congenital, neoplastic* and *inflammatory* lesions of the brain as well as, or better than, CT. It can also define *vascular* lesions such as angiomas, aneurysms, subdural and extradural haematomas (Figs. 12.20, 12.21, 12.22 and 12.23).

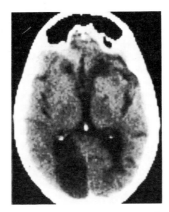

Fig. 12.19   Mature Rt occipital infarct of c.s.f. density like the ventricles (L40 W80).

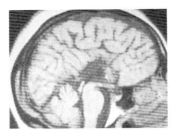

Fig. 12.20   Complete agenesis of the corpus callosum shown by midline sagittal MRI section.

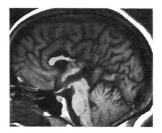

Fig. 12.21 Partial agenesis of the corpus callosum.

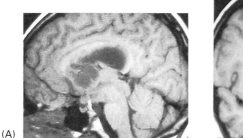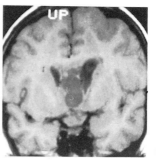

(A) (B)

Fig. 12.22 Glioma involving anterior part of third ventricle and spreading up the septum pellucidum. (A) Sagittal and (B) coronal MRI studies (T_1-weighted) show irregular mass of low signal.

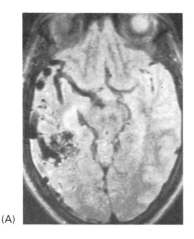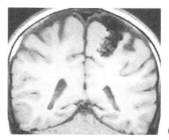

(A) (B)

Fig. 12.23 (A) MR study (T_2-weighted). Right temporoparietal angioma supplied by hypertrophied middle cerebral artery. (B) Coronal MR study (T_1-weighted) of small left parasagittal angioma showing cone-like extension into brain.

MRI is superior to CT in the posterior fossa since the images are not obscured by the dense petrous blocks. Even small acoustic tumours within the internal auditory meatus or just protruding from it can be well shown (Fig. 12.24). MRI is also superior for lesions of the cranio-vertebral junction.

More recently new techniques have made possible *MRI angio-*

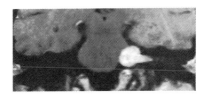

Fig. 12.24   Coronal MRI study (T_1-weighted) after i.v. gadolinium shows high signal from a small acoustic tumour extending into the IAM. Note complete absence of bone image or artefact compared with CT. (Courtesy of Dr Peter Phelp.)

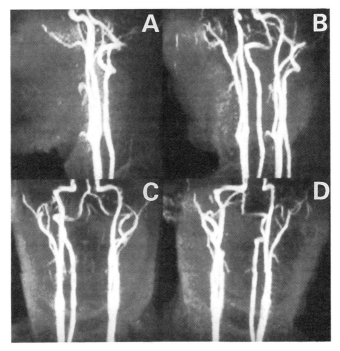

Fig. 12.25   Projection images. (A) Sagittal, (B) LAO, (C) Coronal and (D) RAO planes, from a time-of-flight MR angiogram showing normal neck and basal arteries. (Courtesy of IGE.)

graphy of a quality which is beginning to rival direct angiography and holds the promise of eventually supplanting it (Fig. 12.25).

Lesions of the white matter can be easily shown, and in this respect MRI is more sensitive than CT. The plaques of multiple sclerosis are particularly well shown (Fig. 12.26), as are oedema and other disturbances of the white matter.

Study of the spinal cord is particularly suited to MRI because of the ease of obtaining sagittal sections. Spinal tumours and cystic lesions such as syringomyelia can now be imaged non-invasively and without the necessity for myelography (see below).

Orbits

High resolution images of the orbital contents can now be obtained by MRI and without the radiation hazard involved in CT (Fig. 12.27). This enables most intraorbital masses to be localised and characterised.

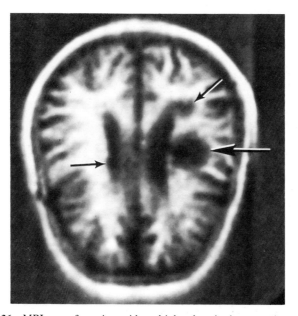

Fig. 12.26 MRI scan of a patient with multiple sclerosis. Arrows point to areas of low density adjacent to the ventricles. The format is similar to a conventional CT scan but there is better differentiation of white and grey matter. Only the large lesion was identified at CT (courtesy of Professor R. Steiner).

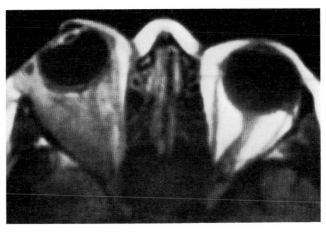

Fig. 12.27 T₁ weighted image showing a diffuse mass in the right orbit due to a pseudotumour. The normal optic nerve is well shown on the left.

THE SPINE AND SPINAL CORD

The methods currently used for investigation of the spine and spinal cord include:

1. Simple X-rays
2. Radioisotopes
3. Myelography and radiculography
4. CT and computed myelography (CM)
5. MRI
6. Spinal angiography.

A plain X-ray of the spine, like a plain X-ray of the skull, will often provide helpful information as to the cause of a neurological disability. *Inflammatory* lesions such as tuberculosis of the spine may be demonstrated, as may *neoplastic* lesions such as secondary deposits involving the bony spine. *Congenital anomalies* may also be demonstrated, and these, particularly in the cervical region, are now being increasingly recognised in association with neurological disorders.

The value of radiology in the diagnosis of fractures and dislocations of the spine is self-evident.

Evidence of *disc lesions* may also be shown by plain X-ray. The importance of *lumbar disc protrusions* as the major cause of sciatica has long been known. The role of the *cervical disc* in the production of brachial neuritis and of pyramidal signs in the elderly is also well recognised. Evidence of these disc lesions is usually present on plain X-ray, but the radiological findings of disc narrowing and adjacent bony sclerosis or lipping must be carefully correlated with the clinical aspects of the problem since disc degeneration without significant symptoms is common in the middle-aged and elderly.

Evidence of the presence of an *intraspinal tumour* may occasionally be seen in a plain X-ray, manifesting itself as erosion of adjacent vertebral pedicles or vertebral body.

Radioisotopes are useful in identifying lesions of the bony spine, particularly multiple metastases and their use in this context has been described above (Ch. 6).

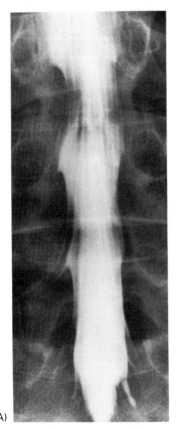 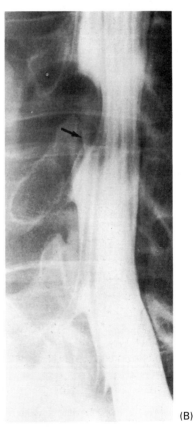

(A)   (B)

Fig. 12.28 Prolapsed L3/4 intervertebral disc. Radiculogram.
A. Anteroposterior. B. Right posterior oblique projections. The disc substance impresses the right anterolateral aspect of the contrast column at L3/4 disc level. The right 3rd lumbar root is compressed against the pedicle of the corresponding vertebra and the 4th lumbar root is deviated medially (→).

Spinal angiography is used for the diagnosis of the rare vascular lesions involving the cord. These include angiomas and dural AV fistulas. It is also diagnostic for the rare haemangioblastoma of the spinal cord.

Myelography and *radiculography* are now performed with water soluble low osmolar contrast media such as Niopam. These can demonstrate both intramedullary and extramedullary tumours affecting the cord and cauda equina. They can also demonstrate disc protrusions (Fig. 12.28).

CT shows bony lesions in greater detail than simple X-ray and will also show disc lesions (Fig. 12.29). However *computed myel-*

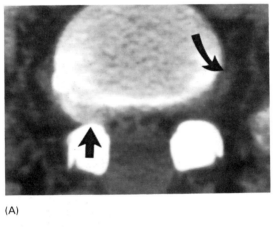

(A)

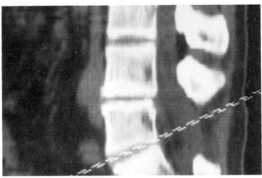

(B)

Fig. 12.29 CT following a laminectomy which failed to cure the patient. There is a large lateral disc herniation occluding the right intervertebral foramen and compressing the right 5th lumbar nerve root (↑). The left root is shown exiting the foramen (↘). (B) shows the plane of section through L5–S1.

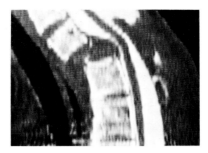

Fig. 12.30 Computed myelogram – reformatted sagittal section. Collapsed vertebra due to neoplasm impinging on theca and cord. Previous laminectomy. The opacified CSF in the subarachnoid space (white) outlines the cord (black).

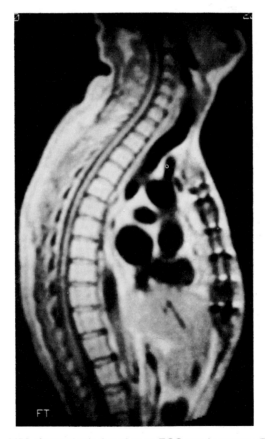

Fig. 12.31 MRI of normal spinal cord on an ECG-gated sequence (ECG SE 1000/24).

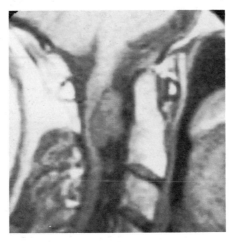

Fig. 12.32 Sagittal MRI study shows ovoid tumour lying anterior to the spinal cord behind C2 (neurofibroma). (Courtesy of Dr J. B. Bradshaw and Bristol Medico-chirurgical Journal.)

ography (CM) is necessary for it to define the spinal cord and most lesions involving it (Fig. 12.30). CM requires the introduction of only a small amount of Niopam by lumbar puncture shortly before examination by CT. It can also performed following a more formal myelogram or radiculogram.

MRI despite its high cost is now the primary investigation of choice in the diagnosis of most lesions affecting the spinal cord and in many lesions affecting the bony spine (Figs 12.31 and 12.32). Intramedullary lesions of the cord are particularly well defined including tumours both solid and cystic. Syringomyelia is also easily diagnosed (Fig. 12.33), and degenerative and inflammatory lesions can be recognised.

MRI also offers a non-invasive method for diagnosing disc protrusions (Fig. 12.34).

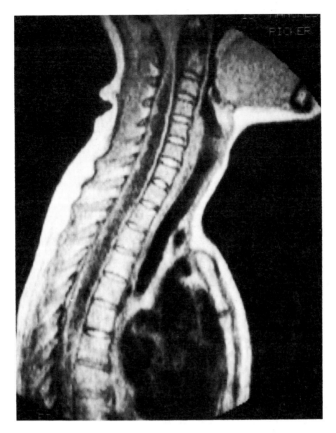

Fig. 12.33 Syringomelia shown on midline MRI sagittal section. The extent of the syrinx cavity and degree of hindbrain herniation are demonstrated. The fourth ventricle (not shown) is in normal position (SE 1000/24).

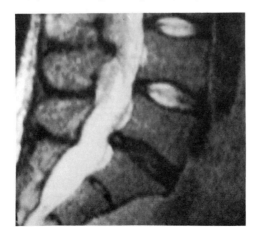

Fig. 12.34 Sagittal MRI section shows normal disc signals at L2–3 and L3–4 but degenerate disc at L4–5 with disc protusion indenting theca.

13. Soft tissues: interventional radiology

SOFT TISSUES

All radiographs have a soft tissue component and it is important to pay due attention to this, though it is often overexposed to show bone detail. If necessary the soft tissues should be examined with a spotlight. Lesions of soft tissues can be better demonstrated by films specially underexposed or by the special techniques of xeroradiography, CT and MRI.

The recognition of opaque *foreign bodies* in the soft tissues was amongst the earliest uses of X-rays. Metallic foreign bodies show up well as do many other types of material. Glass often contains enough lead to render it radiopaque.

Calcification in the soft tissues is not uncommon. Arterial calcification is frequent in the elderly and is usually due to atheroma in the abdominal aorta and iliacs or in the aortic arch. Widespread arterial calcification may be seen in *hyperparathyroidism* when it may be obvious even in peripheral arteries. Other conditions with a high serum calcium such as *chronic renal failure*, particularly with prolonged haemodialysis can give rise to ectopic calcification around joints. *Gout* may also show calcified tophi in the soft tissues and *scleroderma* is frequently associated with calcification in the digits. The rare condition of *dermatomyositis* can give rise to strikingly extensive calcification in the soft tissues.

More common causes of soft tissue calcification are *tuberculous glands* in the neck, mediastinum or abdomen and calcification in *damaged tendons* such as the supraspinatus tendon. It may also occur in *thyroid adenomas* and in a variety of soft tissue tumours both benign and malignant.

Parasitic calcification is described in a wide number of infestations including *cysticercosis* and *guinea worm* when the appearances are characteristic.

Xeroradiography

This is a technique of recording the latent images in a beam of X-rays transmitted through a patient, not as a direct photograph, but as a change in the electrostatic charge in a thin layer of a special plate. The plates are made of selenium which is a good electrical insulator until irradiated when charge carriers are discharged in the irradiated region. The discharge occurs locally leaving the non-irradiated region charged.

The plate is first charged by passing it under a series of corona discharge wires and has a potential of 7000–10 000 volts. The latent image consists of the pattern of the discharge caused by the transmission of an X-ray beam through a patient. This image is usually developed by dusting the selenium surface with fine charged particles. When settled on the plate the powder forms the image. This is made permanent by pressing a paper coated with translucent plastic against the plate. The paper is peeled off taking with it the powder which is then sealed into the plastic surface by heating. The used plate can be repeatedly re-cycled.

The great advantage of xeroradiography is the range of contrast possible. This makes it an ideal method for the examination of soft tissues and in particular, for mammography where it is widely used. Figure 13.1 shows the fine soft tissue detail that is possible.

Xeroradiography is also used for the demonstration of bone lesions, e.g. in the hands where it is desired to see fine detail well. Localisation of foreign bodies of low density is another practical use of the method. It cannot be widely used for the examination of thick parts like the abdomen as the X-ray dosage rates increase very rapidly in such thick parts.

The soft tissues are also well shown by the more expensive imaging techniques of CT and MRI.

MAMMOGRAPHY

Mammography either using conventional radiography or xeroradiography is now widely practised for the investigation of breast lesions and the assessment of suspected breast carcinomas. Breast carcinoma often shows characteristic radiological changes enabling it to be differentiated from benign tumours such as fibroadenomas or from cysts.

Radiological characteristics of a typical carcinoma are high density of the lesion, an irregular margin with spiculation, fine punctate calcification within the lesion, and overlying skin thickening or dimpling, though not all features will necessarily be present in an individual carcinoma (Fig. 13.1). A fibroadenoma is usually smoothly lobulated in outline and calcification if present is denser and coarser than with a carcinoma (Fig. 13.2).

INTERVENTIONAL RADIOLOGY

In many of the previous chapters interventional techniques of

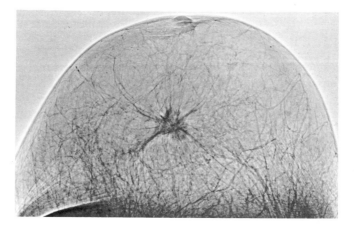

Fig. 13.1 Xeroradiograph showing small spiculated breast carcinoma lying centrally.

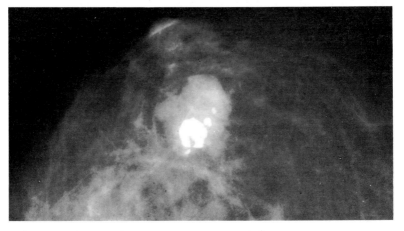

Fig. 13.2 Mammogram using conventional radiography showing fibroadenoma of breast, partially calcified.

radiology have been mentioned. In recent years the number of procedures used by the radiologist not only for diagnosis but for active treatment of the patients have increased. The main procedures used can be classified as follows:

1. Needle biopsies

Fine needle biopsy of many deep seated tumours can now be performed by simple percutaneous puncture by the radiologist with the help of image intensifier screening. The procedure is widely practised for obtaining biopsy material from peripheral nodules in the lung. It can also be used for obtaining bone biopsies from the spine or limbs by percutaneous puncture. The use of this simple technique can prevent an exploratory thoracotomy or other major operation. Fine needle biopsies can also be obtained from retroperitoneal nodes. The development of ultrasound and CT has enabled the method to be extended to formerly inaccessible organs. Ultrasound guided biopsy can be used for kidneys and other abdominal organs. Even greater accuracy of biopsy can be obtained for quite small lesions using CT guidance. If the procedure is done actually on the CT table it is possible to obtain a percutaneous biopsy even from small pancreatic lesions or from other retroperitoneal structures (Fig. 13.3).

2. The biliary tract

Percutaneous puncture of the gall-bladder by a fine needle with aspiration of contents can be performed under ultrasound guidance in patients with acute cholecystitis. The procedure can be combined with antegrade cholecystography to demonstrate the associated cystic duct occlusion (Fig.13.4).

Percutaneous catheter drainage of empyema is also possible using a transhepatic approach (Fig.13.5).

Percutaneous removal of biliary duct stones. A major problem in the biliary tract is the patient with stones in the ducts which have not been found at operation and are later demonstrated by postoperative T-tube cholangiography. It is possible for the radiologist to remove such stones and save the patient from a further laparotomy. A guide wire is inserted into the ducts through the T-tube tract and a catheter with a wire snare is passed over the guide wire and into the ducts. The stones can then be snared and removed through the T-tube tract.

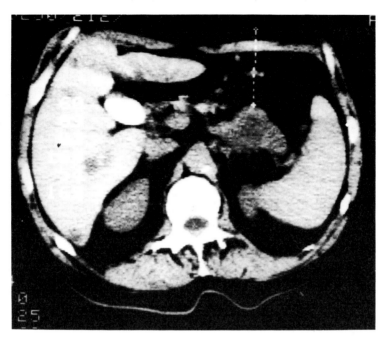

Fig. 13.3 Percutaneous fine needle biopsy of small pancreatic tumour in the pancreatic tail. The tumour lies 6 cm from the skin surface as shown on the electronic guideline. The low density lesions in the liver are metastases.

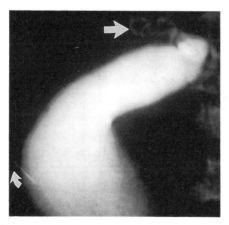

Fig. 13.4 Antegrade cholecystogram performed under ultrasound guidance with 22 swg needle (curved arrow). Note calculi in the cystic duct (arrow). (Courtesy of Dr W. R. Lees.)

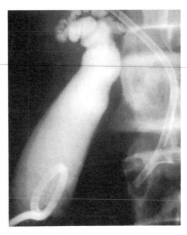

Fig. 13.5 Empyema secondary to endoscopic stenting for biliary malignancy. A locking pigtail catheter is inserted to provide long-term drainage. The stent in the CBD is also shown. (Courtesy of Dr. W. R. Lees.)

Percutaneous biliary duct drainage. Patients with obstructive jaundice can, as described in Chapter 9, be investigated by fine needle percutaneous cholangiography. Once the dilated ducts have been demonstrated these can also be catheterised percutaneously and a drain left *in situ* to decompress the biliary system and relieve the patient's acute symptoms.

Percutaneous insertion of bypass prosthesis. In some of these cases, which are usually due to carcinoma near the lower·end of the common bile duct, it is possible using a similar technique to that just described to pass a small prosthesis through the stricture. This provides internal drainage for the lesion permitting a more comfortable terminal stage for the patient and considerable relief of symptoms.

Endoscopic sphincterotomy can be performed using diathermy introduced through the endoscope and following endoscopic cholangiograpy to show stones or stricture. The stones can then be removed immediately using a balloon or basket passed through the endoscope (Fig.13.6). Alternatively the stones can be left to pass naturally through the widened sphincter. In the case of stricture a stent can be inserted retrogradely via the endoscope.

3. The portal system

Percutaneous trans-hepatic embolisation of varices. As noted in a previous chapter the portal system can be investigated by percu-

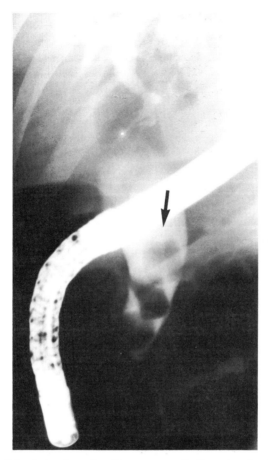

Fig. 13.6 Following endoscopic sphincterotomy, a balloon-tipped catheter has been passed down the endoscope and into the duct. The balloon is inflated (arrow) above the stones and traction delivers the stones into the duodenum.

taneous trans-hepatic catheterisation of the portal veins. Once varices have been demonstrated by this method it is possible to manipulate the tip of the catheter into the main drainage veins of the varices and to percutaneously embolise them.

Percutaneous venous sampling for APUD tumours. Using the same technique of percutaneous catheterisation of the portal vein, venous samples can be obtained at various sites along the course of the splenic vein and its branches which can help considerably in localising small insulinomas or other pancreatic endocrine tumours.

4. Haemorrhage

Upper GI haemorrhage is a major problem in hospital practice. Most patients who are in fairly good condition will be investigated by endoscopy. Others who are severely shocked and bleeding rapidly may require emergency laparotomy. An intermediate group of cases and those in whom endoscopy has failed to demonstrate a lesion can be further investigated by angiography and treated at the same time. To demonstrate the bleed by angiography the patient must be actually bleeding at the time of investigation. The angiogram will then show escape of contrast at the point of the bleed, whether this is a Mallory–Weiss tear at the lower end of the oesophagus, or a peptic ulcer in the stomach or duodenum. Haemorrhage can be controlled in these cases by intra-arterial infusion of vasopressin or by embolisation. Haemorrhage from varices has been mentioned above and can be controlled by transhepatic portal phlebography and embolisation.

Persistent haemorrhage from the colon or lower small bowel can also be investigated by angiography. This is usually due to haemorrhage from an area of angiodysplasia or from a colonic diverticulum. The lesion must be demonstrated angiographically before surgery can be effective since such lesions are notoriously difficult to find at laparotomy.

Pelvic haemorrhage may be difficult to control in carcinoma of the bladder or cervix, or in a post irradiation or post-traumatic situation. Such haemorrhage can be effectively treated by embolisation of the internal iliacs or their branches.

Renal haemorrhage from neoplasm or trauma can also be treated by superselective embolisation (Fig. 13.7) as can hepatic haemorrhage.

The method has also been used in severe epistaxis and in bleeding from head and neck neoplasms and in severe haemoptysis.

5. The urinary tract

Antegrade nephrostomy by percutaneous needle puncture or catheterisation has been mentioned above. The percutaneous insertion of a drainage catheter into the opacified pelvis can be a very valuable procedure in these cases as a preliminary to operation and for diagnostic purposes (Fig. 13.8). The same route can be used for *the introduction of stents* or *dilatation of ureteric strictures*. *Percutaneous stone removal* is also possible from the catheter tract.

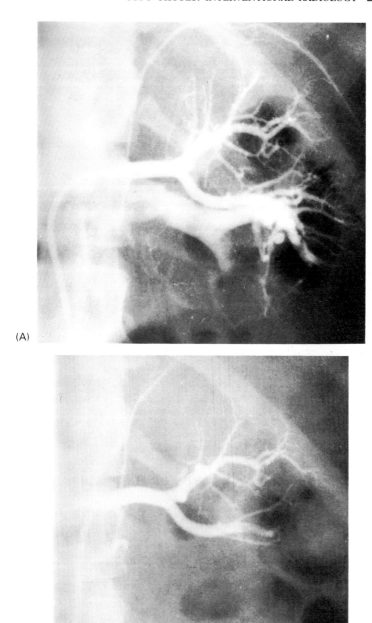

(A)

(B)

Fig. 13.7   (A) Renal AV fistula following renal biopsy. (B) Same case after embolisation of fistula.

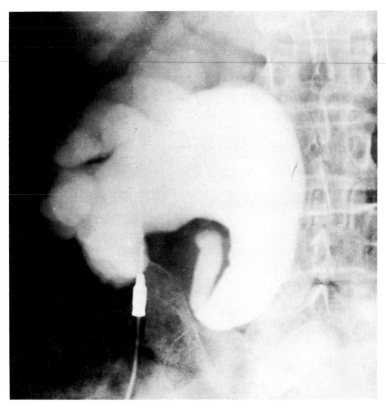

Fig. 13.8   Antegrade nephrostomy. A needle has been inserted into an upper calyx from the back and contrast injected. This facilitates introduction of a percutaneous catheter.

Renal cyst puncture can be done percutaneously, preferably under ultrasound control. Large cysts can be drained though they do tend to recur, usually after a few years. Permanent cure can be obtained by insertion of a sclerosant towards the end of the drainage procedure.

6. Percutaneous embolisation of tumours

Following selective percutaneous angiography highly vascular tumours can be embolised using Gelfoam, Butylacrilate (an instant setting polymer adhesive), steel coils and various other foreign bodies. The methods have proved extremely valuable as a pre-operative measure with highly vascular tumours or as an alternative measure where surgical excision is considered impossible or

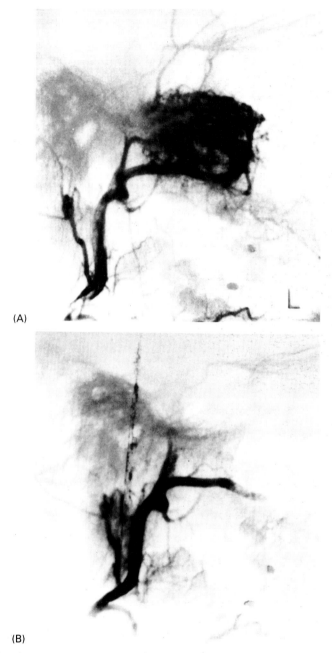

(A)

(B)

Fig. 13.9 Juvenile angiofibroma of nasopharynx. (A) Before. (B) After embolisation. The internal maxillary artery has been superselectively catheterised.

difficult, or if there is a relative contraindication to surgery such as severe ischaemia or respiratory disease. The method is extremely useful in the vascular juvenile angiofibroma, a tumour which occurs in the nasopharynx of adolescent males (Fig. 13.9). It is also useful in glomus jugulare tumours and has been used in vascular meningiomas. The method has also been used in hypernephromas and in malignant liver tumours.

7. Percutaneous embolisation of angiomas, arteriovenous (AV) fistula, and aneurysm

The technique of percutaneous catheter embolisation has also been widely used for the treatment of angiomatous malformations, particularly in the distribution of the external carotid artery (Fig. 13.10). AV fistula has also been treated by this technique. Carotico-cavernous and even vertebral AV fistula have also

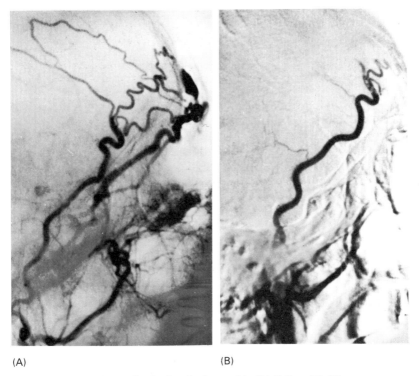

(A)   (B)

Fig. 13.10   Angioma of scalp directly above orbit. (A) Before. (B) After embolisation of superficial temporal artery supply.

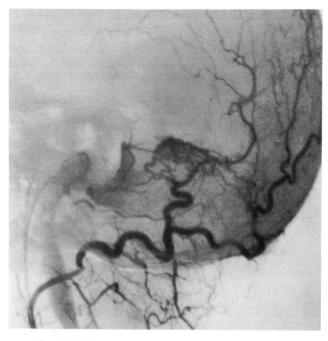

Fig. 13.11   Dural AV fistula supplied by the occipital artery and draining into the lateral sinus and internal jugular vein. Superselective occipital artery injection (subtraction print). This case was successfully treated by percutaneous embolisation.

been cured by a modification of the technique. These latter lesions have been treated with an ingenious detachable balloon introduced by percutaneous catheter. Dural AV fistula has also been successfully treated by embolisation (Fig. 13.11), as have aneurysms.

8. Percutaneous angioplasty

It is now possible for the radiologist to treat severe arterial stenosis and even an occlusion in the iliac and femoral arteries by passing a guide wire through the lesion followed by a catheter with an inflatable balloon. This dilates up the diseased segment and can restore good arterial flow without the necessity for an open operation. The technique has also been used on stenosed renal arteries and, in a modified form, even on coronaries in carefully selected cases. Figure 13.12 shows an iliac artery before and after a percutaneous dilatation with a Gruntzig balloon catheter.

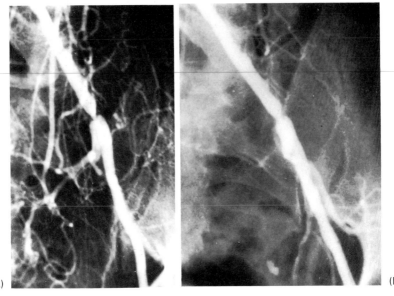

Fig. 13.12 Gruntzig catheter dilatation of arterial stenosis. (A) Before. (B) After.

(A)   (B)

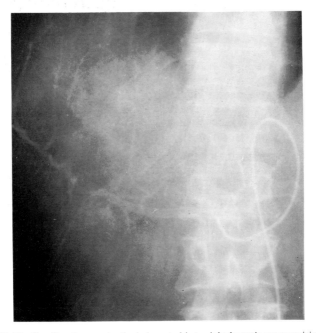

Fig. 13.13 Small catheter selectively inserted into right hepatic artery arising from superior mesenteric artery. The catheter was left in situ for several days for infusion of cytotoxic drugs. Multiple liver secondaries. The site confirmed by contrast injection.

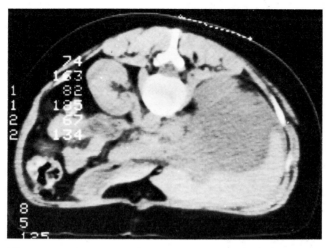

(A)

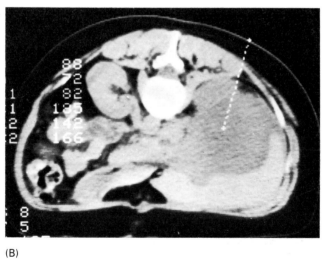

(B)

Fig. 13.14 CT scans of prone patient showing a large right subhepatic abscess, secondary to GB surgery. Electronic cursors are used to measure (A) distance from midline to avoid kidney (B) distance to centre of abscess.

In recent years angioplasty has also become possible using rotating cams or lasers, and intra-arterial stents have been used to maintain patency.

9. Intra-arterial chemotherapy and thrombolysis

Maximal therapeutic doses of cytotoxic drugs may be delivered directly to tumours by selective arterial catheterisation. The technique has been used for inoperable tumours, particularly liver metastases (Fig. 13.13) and for the treatment of large malignant tumours.

A similar technique is used for the treatment of acute embolic or thrombotic occlusions by streptokinase or tissue plasmogen activator (TPA).

10. Percutaneous abscess drainage

Intra-abdominal and other deep-seated abscesses, particularly post-operative, can now be accurately diagnosed and localised by ultrasound or CT, which can then be used to guide the percutaneous insertion of a drain. This technique has revolutionised the treatment of such lesions by providing a safer and simpler alternative to laparotomy in seriously ill patients (Fig. 13.14 A and B).

Index